WN 230 POR

OXFORD MEDICAL PUBLICATIONS

RADIOGRAPHIC INTERPRETATION
IN OROFACIAL DISEASE

Radiographic Interpretation in Orofacial Disease

·

EDITED BY

STEPHEN R. PORTER

*Honorary Lecturer, University Department of
Oral Medicine, Surgery, and Pathology,
Bristol, UK*

AND

CRISPIAN SCULLY

*Professor, University Department of
Oral Medicine, Surgery, and Pathology,
Bristol, UK*

Oxford   New York   Tokyo
OXFORD UNIVERSITY PRESS
1991

Oxford University Press, Walton Street, Oxford OX2 6DP

Oxford New York Toronto
Delhi Bombay Calcutta Madras Karachi
Petaling Jaya Singapore Hong Kong Tokyo
Nairobi Dar es Salaam Cape Town
Melbourne Auckland

and associated companies in
Berlin Ibadan

Oxford is a trade mark of Oxford University Press

Published in the United States
by Oxford University Press, New York

British Library Cataloguing in Publication Data
Radiographic interpretation in orofacial disease.
1. Dentistry. Diagnosis. Radiography
I. Porter, Stephen R.   II. Scully, C. M. (Crispian
Michael)
617.60757
ISBN 0–19–261585–8

Library of Congress Cataloging in Publication Data
Radiographic interpretation of orofacial disease / edited by
Stephen R. Porter and Crispian Scully.
p.   cm.—(Oxford medical publications)
1. Teeth—Radiography.   2. Mouth—Radiography.   3. Jaws—
Radiography.   I. Porter, Stephen R.   II. Scully, Crispian.
III. Series.
[DNLM: 1. Stomatognathic System—radiography—problems.   WN 18
R12905]
RK301.R284   1991   617.5'2207572—dc20   90–14165
ISBN 0–19–261585–8

Typeset and Printed by
Butler & Tanner Ltd, Frome and London

PREFACE

RADIOLOGICAL investigations are often undertaken to supplement the history and physical examination to help diagnosis and assess the management of orofacial disorders. It is thus hardly surprising that radiographic interpretation is an almost ubiquitous component in the academic assessment of clinical undergraduates and postgraduates. Many students, however, have limited experience in the analysis of radiographs; indeed for some their first opportunity to examine the radiographs of certain disorders is at the time of their academic examination.

In an attempt to prepare candidates for routine clinical practice and for such examinations we have prepared a selection of radiographs of orofacial disorders.

There are five sections, each containing a spectrum of problems requiring a depth of knowledge that ranges from undergraduate to postgraduate. The information is *not* intended to be comprehensive and should be used to complement standard texts. We appreciate that some clinical problems can be managed in a variety of ways, but the answers given generally reflect the treatment policies of the various institutions with which we have been associated.

Bristol   S.R.P.
1991   C.S.

ACKNOWLEDGEMENTS

MOST of the radiographs used are from our collection and for this our greatest debt is to the patients and referring practitioners.

We are also grateful to the late Professor Arthur Darling and Professor J. Fletcher for use of some radiographs from the Bristol collection; Professor Nairn Wilson and Miss Ann Shearer (Manchester Dental School) for the original loan of radiograph 3.9, Dr John Rayne (Oxford) for use of radiograph 1.7, Dr Jane Luker (Bristol) for 3.3 and Mr John Bunn (Bristol) for 2.7 and 4.10. Nye Fathers and Derek Coles kindly helped with the preparation of the radiographs. We are grateful to Mr Philip Sugerman for useful discussion and comment regarding the manuscript. We are also extremely grateful to Connie Blake for her patience in the typing of the manuscript and to Karen Porter for her help in checking the text.

We are immensely grateful for the assistance and advice of John Bunn and Margaret Lane regarding the many practical aspects of radiology, and to the staff of Oxford University Press who have encouraged and advised us and been responsible for pursuing the book to completion. We thank Heinemann Professional Publishing Ltd. for permission to reproduce some illustrations from *The Dental Patient* and *The Mouth in Health and Disease*.

CONTRIBUTORS

STEPHEN R. PORTER
Honorary Lecturer in Oral Medicine, Surgery and Pathology,
University Department of Oral Medicine, Surgery and Pathology, Bristol, UK

CRISPIAN SCULLY
Professor of Oral Medicine, Surgery and Pathology,
University Department of Oral Medicine, Surgery and Pathology, Bristol, UK

CHRISTOPHER D. STEPHENS
Professor of Child Dental Health,
University Department of Child Dental Health, Bristol, UK

MARK J. GRIFFITHS
Consultant in Oral Medicine and Surgery,
University Department of Oral Medicine, Surgery and Pathology, Bristol, UK

JONATHAN SHEPHERD
Reader in Oral and Maxillo-facial Surgery,
University Department of Oral Medicine, Surgery and Pathology, Bristol, UK

JACK W. ROSS
Consultant in Oral and Maxillo-facial Surgery,
University Department of Oral Medicine, Surgery and Pathology, Bristol, UK

PAPER 1 · QUESTIONS

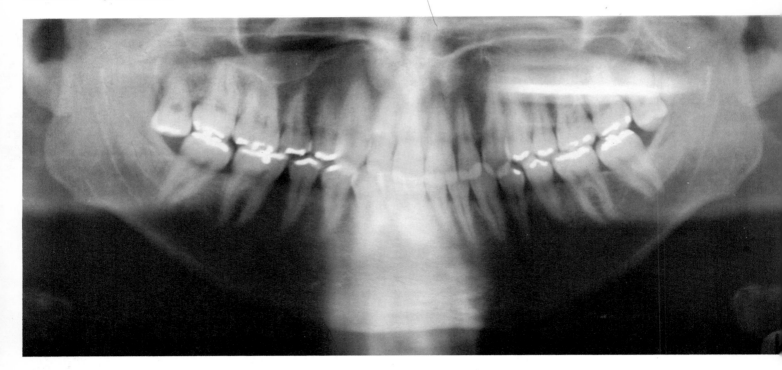

Q1.1   This is a 37 year old haemophiliac.
(a) What oral surgery is needed?
(b) List the possible complications of surgery in this patient and how these can be prevented or managed.

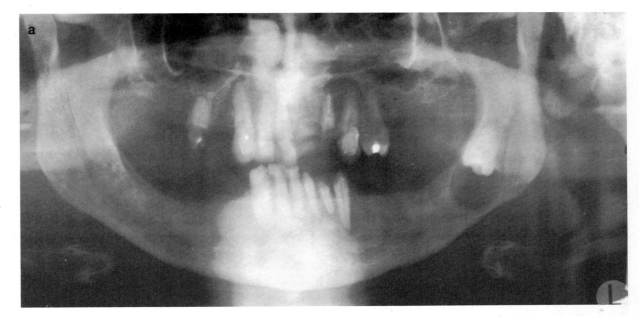

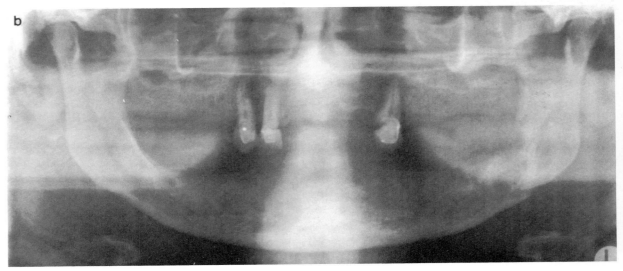

Q1.2 (a) What type of cyst is shown in $\overline{8}$ region in (a)?
(b) Where is the inferior alveolar nerve in (a)?
(c) What does the six-month post-operative radiograph (b) show?

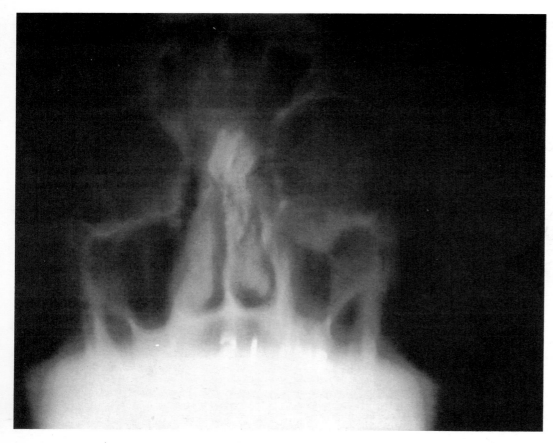

Q1.3   This tomogram shows the maxillo-facial injuries that resulted from a motorcycle accident.
(a) What bony injury is shown?
(b) What consequent soft tissue derangement is shown?

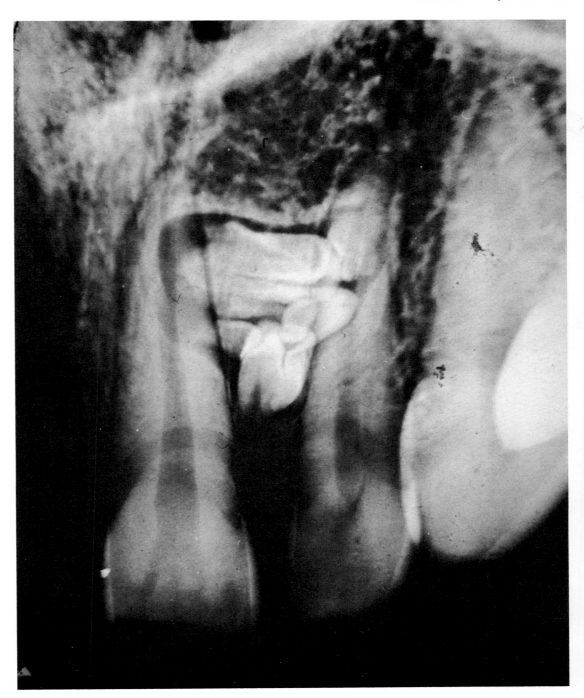

Q1.4   This 12 year old patient complained of a lump on her gum.
(a) Provide a probable diagnosis.
(b) Where do these lesions usually arise?
(c) In which systemic disorder can these lesions often occur?

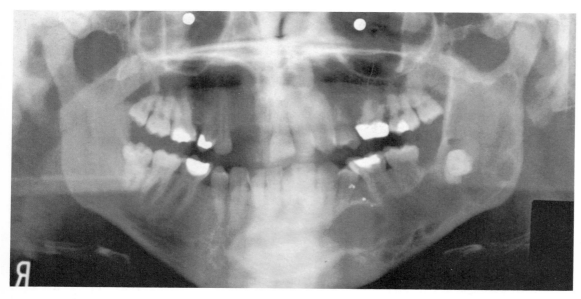

Q1.5   This is the pantomograph of a 35 year old patient.
(a) What is the likely diagnosis of the lesion in the left mandible and what methods
of diagnosis can be applied?
(b) What would be the treatment?

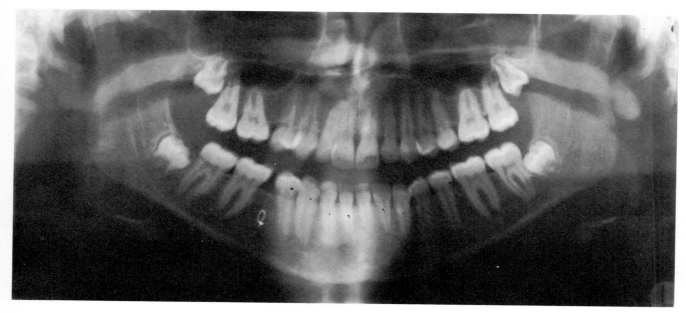

Q1.6   (a) Which teeth are missing?
(b) How might the radio-opaque object mesial to $\overline{6|}$ have achieved its present position,
assuming it is in the alveolus?

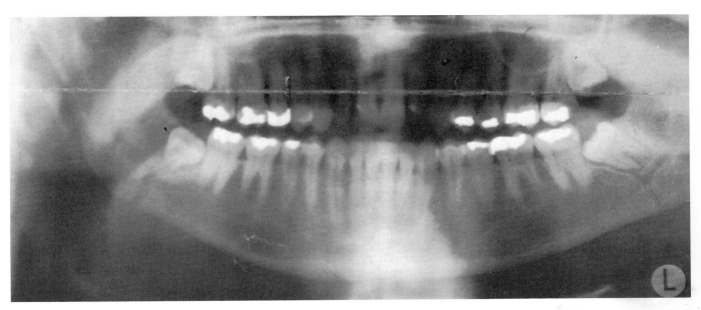

Q1.7   (a) In the days immediately following a road traffic accident, this patient noticed that his teeth did not meet correctly—why?
         (b) What is the management?

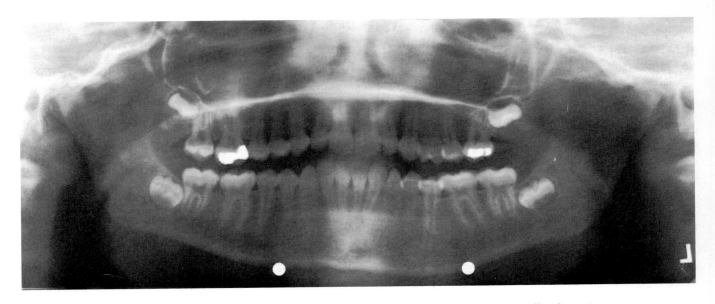

Q1.8   (a) Was the upper left first molar extracted or congenitally absent?
         (b) What is unusual about the pattern of dental caries in this patient?

hypoplastic
caries free

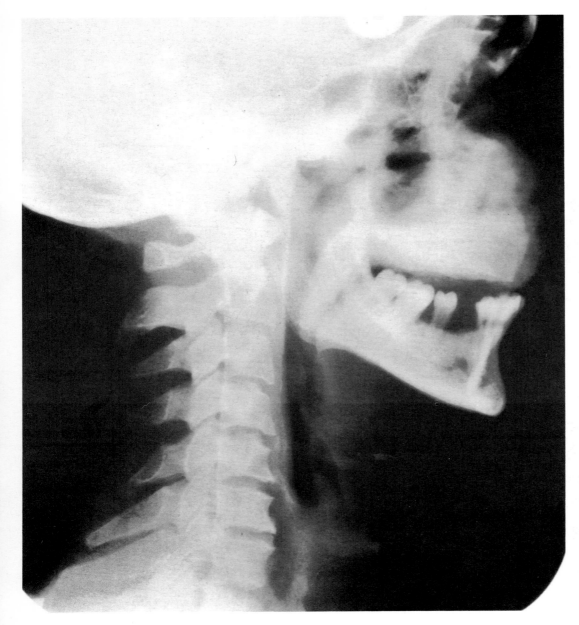

Q1.9 This elderly gentleman complained that his upper lip was becoming more prominent.
(a) Suggest a diagnosis.
(b) What additional investigations will help to confirm the diagnosis?
(c) List the orofacial manifestations of this disorder.

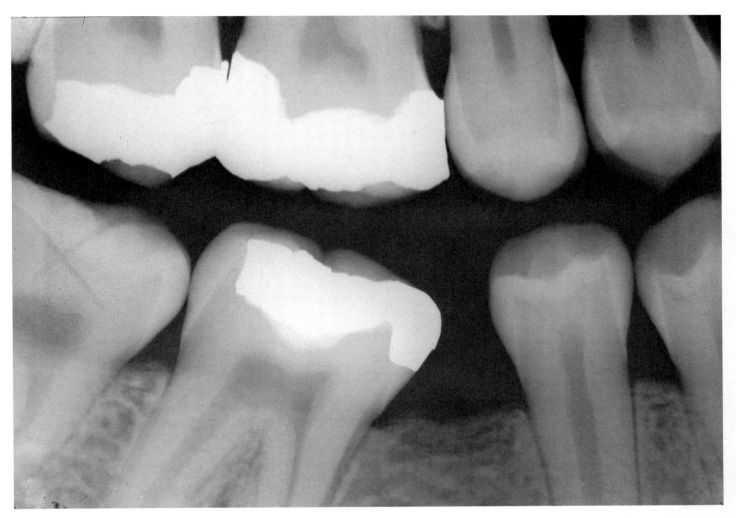

Q1.10   This is a medically fit 21 year old female.
(a) Provide a diagnosis.
(b) Provide a treatment plan.

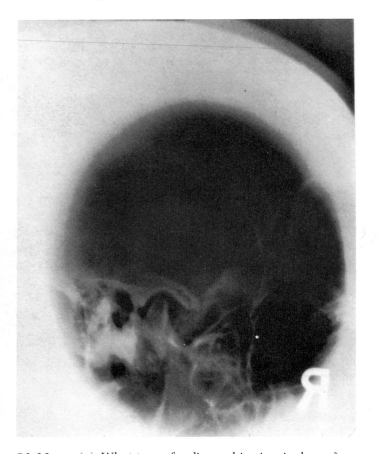 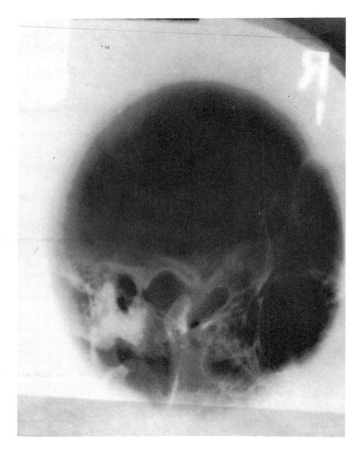

Q1.11   (a) What type of radiographic view is shown?
         (b) What other radiographic investigations of the temporomandibular joint are avail-
              able?

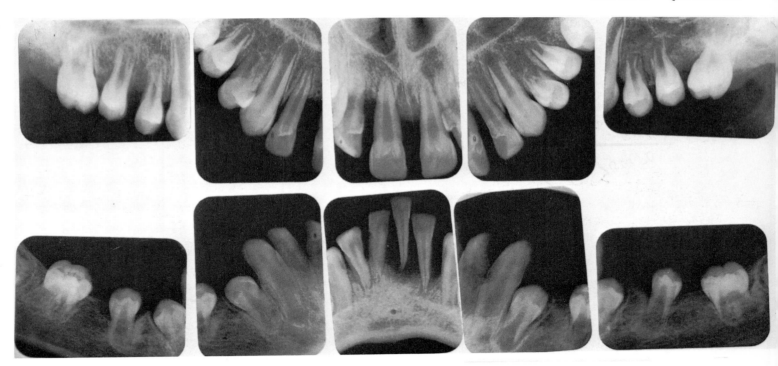

Q1.12 This 9 year old boy has had severe periodontitis since he was 3 years of age.
(a) What type of periodontitis does he have?
(b) The patient has keratotic lesions on his palms and soles of feet. What is the probable diagnosis?

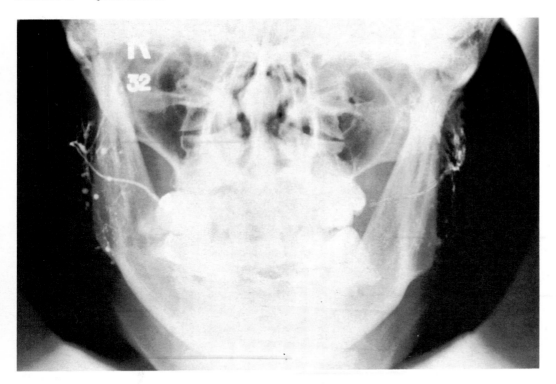

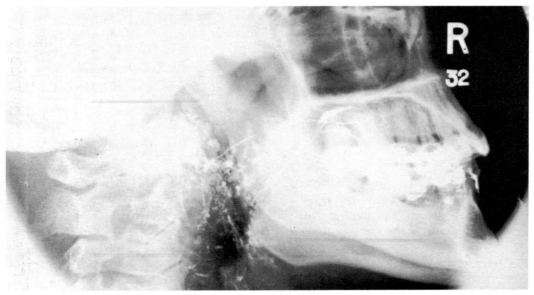

Q1.13   (a) What is this radiological investigation?
(b) What is the abnormality shown and in which disorders is it most likely to occur?
(c) What other salivary lesions can be detected using this technique?
(d) What non-radiological technique occasionally permits localization of parotid abscesses?

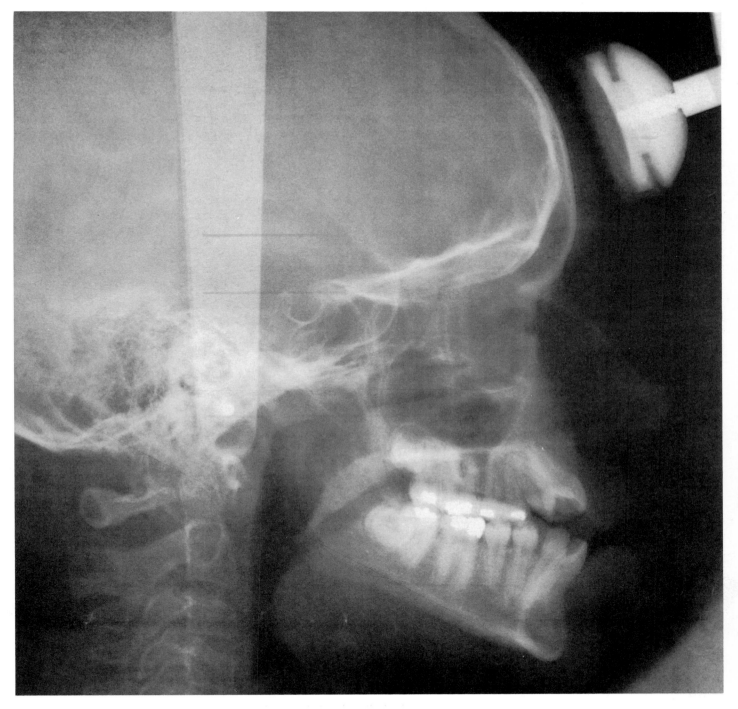

Q1.14   (a) Give an assessment of this patient's lateral skull radiograph.
                 (b) What is the likely cause of the anterior open bite?

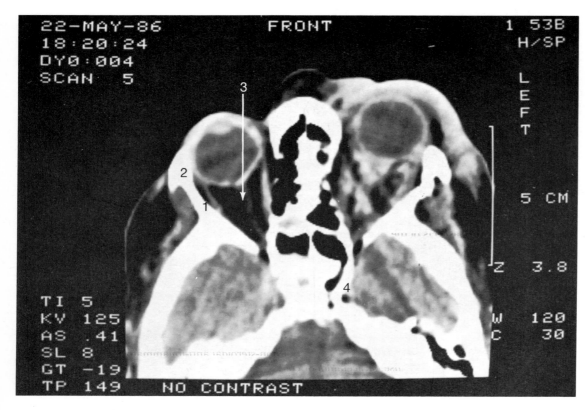

Q1.15 (a) What are structures 1–4?

(b) Suggest possible applications of computerized tomography (CT) in the diagnosis of oral disease.

PAPER 1 · ANSWERS

A1.1   (a) Removal of over-erupted <u>8|8</u>.

        (b) Bleeding:

            (i) Check <u>coagulation state.</u>

            (ii) Give <u>Factor VIII pre-operatively</u>.

            (iii) Desmopressin (DDAVP) therapy may also help.

            (iv) Avoid raising mucoperiosteal flap—this minimizes bleeding into fascial spaces.

            (v) Post-operative tranexamic acid (1 g 4 times a day) can minimize any fibrinolytic tendency.

            (vi) Possible risk from viral carriage or other aspects.

Table A1.1   Other aspects of the management of haemophilia

HIV risk Hepatitis B, C, or D risk Drug addiction	Treat as inoculation risk
Anxiety	Reassurance Possible use of sedation
Drug-induced bleeding	Avoid aspirin and most non-steroidal anti-inflammatory drugs; use paracetamol or codeine phosphate instead

A1.2   (a) Dentigerous cyst.

        (b) The mandibular canal and the inferior alveolar nerve have been displaced downwards and lie close to the inferior border of the mandible. In this position the nerve is relatively unlikely to be damaged, unless there is vigorous curettage of the cyst lining. In this particular case a small amount of <u>mental paraesthesia</u> occurred following enucleation of the cyst.

            A postero-anterior (PA) view of the mandible is advisable before surgery to confirm the relative position of the teeth, cyst, and canal and to estimate the thickness of the bone medially and laterally.

        (c) There has been good healing in the lower left third molar region. There is evidence of new bone formation in the former cyst areas, the outlines of which are becoming less clear as blood vessels grow in. The appearance of the lower border of the mandible suggests that a fracture has occurred but this is another example of the need for a <u>full transmission view such as a lateral oblique mandible</u>.

            A small portion of the apex of the lower left third molar root has been retained.

A1.3   (a) There is fracture and displacement of the nasal septum, nasal bones, and frontal sinuses. There is a defect in the left orbital floor such that soft tissue has protruded into the antrum ('<u>orbital blow-out</u>').

        (b) As a result of entrapment of soft tissue the eye was unable to rotate upwards and the patient had <u>double vision in the upper fields.</u>

        It was previously believed that the entrapment included the inferior rectus or inferior oblique muscle necessarily, but recent work has shown that it is <u>the radial fibrous septum in the orbit</u> that may be <u>trapped and cause limitation</u> of movement of the eyeball.

A1.4   (a) This is a <u>compound odontome</u>.

(b) Compound composite odontomes usually occur in the maxillary canine/incisor region. In contrast, complex odontomes have a more irregular appearance and particularly occur in the molar regions.

(c) Gardner's syndrome (familial adenomatosis coli). This is an autosomal dominant disorder characterized by:

Adenomatous polyposis of the colon (which often leads to colonic carcinoma)
Desmoid tumours
Multiple osteomas of the jaws
Impacted teeth
Supernumerary teeth
Compound odontomes.

Dental anomalies may be seen in up to 30 per cent of affected individuals and often there is a correlation between the presence of dental abnormalities and the number of osteomas. Dentists may thus be the first clinicians to detect affected individuals.

A1.5
(a) The lesion extends from the condylar neck to the $\overline{3}$ region. Presence of buried teeth within the cyst is suggestive of a possible diagnosis of a dentigerous cyst and this was made more likely by aspiration of the cyst fluid, which showed cholesterol crystals. If the cyst had been a keratocyst, aspiration might have been difficult or impossible because of the keratin contained in the cyst. Total protein examination of the aspirate would not establish the diagnosis but would show if protein was at a lower level than 4 g/100 ml.

There is also the possibility that this could be an ameloblastoma because of its position in the mandible and the suspicion of locules in one of the margins. Histopathology provides the definitive diagnosis.

Another possible diagnosis is an odontogenic myxoma, which being a solid tumour could not be aspirated.

(b) The cyst was enucleated via an intra-oral approach and the tooth removed.

The cyst was attached around the neck of the tooth, thus supporting a diagnosis of dentigerous cyst. There was no pre-operative mental anaesthesia and although the nerve had been pushed aside by the cyst it was possible to enucleate the cyst without damage to the nerve.

A1.6
(a) $\frac{5}{3}$ are absent.

(b) This is an orthodontic separating wire that became lodged in the lower second deciduous molar socket when this tooth was removed before molar bands were placed.

A1.7
(a) There are bilateral fractures of the body of the mandible running through the sockets of the impacted lower third molars.

(b) Reduction and immobilization of the fractures will be required because there is occlusal derangement. In addition, the fractures should be assumed to be compound as the unerupted lower third permanent molars are probably in communication with the mouth, and thus systemic antibiotic therapy is required.

In most instances, partially erupted or unerupted third molars do not cause difficulties, indeed, they can help immobilize fractures. However, these teeth should be removed if they prevent adequate fracture reduction or if there is severe pericoronitis.

In view of the adequate complement of healthy teeth in this case, eyelet wires with intermaxillary wires should provide adequate immobilization. Alternatively, arch bars could be used; they have the advantage of allowing elastic bands to be easily placed if the intermaxillary fixation has to be prematurely removed. Plates are becoming a popular means of providing fixation as they avoid the need for intermaxillary fixation and allow good apposition of fragments.

Haemophilia 1 Check coagulation state nt molars is extremely rare. Two radiographic
2 Factor VIII preoperatively. n here.
3 Desmopressin therapy.   ggesting that this tooth has tipped mesially at
        ment. If the first molar had been congenitally
         nothing to retain the second molar, which
        liately posterior to |E .
        hence it is likely that the upper left first molar

        les-resistant mouth. The lower arch is caries
        early mesial cavity in |7. Surprisingly |6 has
        ely restored. It is very unusual to see more
        in the lower arch. A possible explanation is
        poplastic. ✗

A1.9   (a) There are 'woolly' radio-opaque lesions causing enlargement and distortion of the
       maxilla. The diagnosis is Paget's disease of bone (osteitis deformans).

       (b) (i) *Biochemistry:*
            Raised serum alkaline phosphatase levels
            Normal serum levels of calcium and phosphate (usually)
            Increased levels of urinary hydroxyproline.

         (ii) *Biopsy:* The histopathological features of Paget's disease vary according to the
            stage of the disease. However, lesions commonly consist of large areas of dense
            sclerotic bone with many haematoxylin-staining reversal lines giving rise to
            a mosaic-like pattern. There are adjacent areas of cellular and vascular fibrous
            tissue with osteoclasts lying within Howship's lacunae and elsewhere. Within
            the fibrous tissue there are osteoblasts laying down new bone. Hyper-
            cementosis (with reversal lines) of adjacent teeth may also be seen.

       (c) (i) Symmetrical enlargement of the maxillary and malar regions.
         (ii) Symmetrical widening of alveolar arches.
         (iii) Loss of lamina dura, root resorption and hypercementosis in adjacent teeth.
         (iv) Spacing of teeth, malocclusion.
         (v) Cranial nerve palsies.
      (vi) In the osteolytic phase there may be excessive post-extraction bleeding. In
            the sclerotic phase there is a susceptibility to post-extraction osteomyelitis.
         (vii) Osteosarcoma is a rare complication.

A.1.10   (a) (i) 'Early' carious lesion on the mesial aspect of 5|.
         (ii) Overhanging amalgam restoration on the mesial aspect of 7|.
         (iii) Absent 6| due to exodontia.
         (iv) Mild periodontal bone loss in $\frac{45|}{45|}$ areas.

       (b) (i) Without previous radiographs it is difficult to determine the progressive
            nature of the carious lesion. Nevertheless, as there is negligible darkening of
            the associated amelo-dentinal junction, removal of the affected tissue is *not*
            justified. Instead a programme of improved oral hygiene care, fluorides, and
            dietary control is required. The lack of any contact point between premolars
            should help minimize further plaque accumulation in this site. This treatment
            should also prevent further periodontal destruction.

(ii) Modification or careful replacement of the restoration in 7|.

(iii) Regular radiographic monitoring of 5|—there is *no* other proven reliable way of assessing an early carious lesion. Due consideration must be given to avoiding excessive radiation exposure of the patient.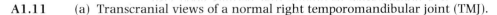

A1.11   (a) Transcranial views of a normal right temporomandibular joint (TMJ).

(b) *Other plain radiographic views:*

  (i)   Transpharyngeal (Toller) views.

  (ii) Townes and reverse Townes views. These are often an adjunct to transcranial or transpharyngeal views as they allow examination of the TMJ in a second plane.

  (iii) Trans-orbital (Zimmer) views—these should not be taken because damage to the eye may occur as a result of the antero-posterior direction of the X-rays.

Tomography:
This allows images of cuts as thin as 1.2 mm to be obtained, but blurring is invariable and the lateral aspects of the TMJ can be particularly difficult to visualize accurately. Nevertheless it is a useful technique when investigating severe fractures of the mandibular condyle or neoplasia in and around the TMJ

    Pantomography—is simple and a convenient way of examining the TMJ but distortion can occur as in any tomograph. Reverse pantomography is better.

Arthrography:
Unlike the aforementioned techniques arthography allows visualization of non-osseous elements such as the joint spaces and the meniscus. A radio-opaque dye—usually iodine-based—is injected into the joint spaces and radiographs or tomographs (arthrotomography) taken at different stages of mouth opening and closing (Fig. A1.11). Newer techniques allow cycles of opening and closing to

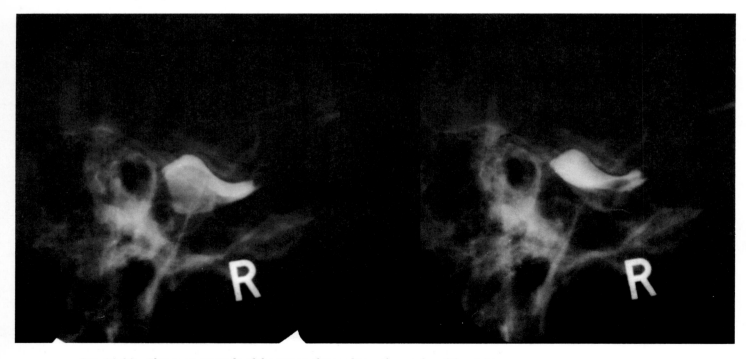

Fig. A1.11   This is an example of the image obtained in arthography of the right temporomandibular joint.

be recorded on videotape, thus the clinician and radiologist can examine joint dynamics in some detail.

Arthography or arthrotomography require sedation of the patient and local analgesia of the skin superficial to the joint.

Computed tomography (CT):
CT is a non-invasive technique that permits good visualization of osseous and non-osseous structures in and about the TMJ. It is mainly used in the investigation of severe TMJ trauma and neoplasia. CT is rarely used in the investigation of TMJ dysfunction syndrome because perforations of the meniscus are difficult to detect (arthrotomography is probably better).

Magnetic resonance imaging (MRI):
The suitability of MRI in the investigation of TMJ disease is still not fully known, but non-osseous elements of the TMJ can be easily visualized. Indeed, in one recent study, abnormalities of the lateral pterygoid muscle and meniscus could reliably be detected by MRI. As MRI is both non-invasive and free of the dangers of ionizing radiation, it is likely to have application in the investigation of TMJ disease.

A1.12 (a) Pre-pubertal periodontitis.

(b) Papillon–Lefevre syndrome (PLS)

This is a rare autosomal recessive disorder. PLS is characterized by severe periodontitis affecting the deciduous and permanent dentitions, and red, scaly, keratotic lesions symmetrically affecting the skin of the dorsal and palmar surfaces of the hands and dorsal and plantar aspects of the feet. Affected individuals occasionally also have an increased susceptibility to infection and to calcification of the tentoria.

The precise cause of the periodontal disease is unknown: the microflora of periodontitis lesions in PLS includes Capnocytophaga, *Actinobacillus actino-mycetemcomitans* and *Bacteroides melaninogenicus* ss. *intermedius,* all of which have tissue-damaging capabilities. A few patients have been found to have diminished neutrophil and/or monocyte function, and cell-mediated immunity may also be mildly defective. Altered ectodermal and/or mesodermal development or collagen metabolism have also been cited as possible causes of PLS. The periodontal disease can be somewhat controlled by conventional measures while the skin lesions can be managed with vitamin A analogues

A1.13 (a) Sialography of the parotid glands. A radio-opaque medium (e.g., an iodine-containing compound such as diatrizoate, iothalamate, or iodinated unsaturated fatty acids) is passed into the duct of the parotid gland. Standard postero-anterior and lateral skull radiographs are taken when the gland is being filled and emptied. Both parotids have been examined here.

(b) There is pooling of contrast medium in dilated ducts and acini, i.e., sialectasis. This is probably due to Sjögren's syndrome but there are other causes (see below).

(c) Sialography can aid the diagnosis of several other salivary disorders; these are summarized in Table A.13.

(d) Very occasionally ultrasonography has been used to investigate parotid lesions—usually abscesses. In this technique high-frequency sound waves pass through the tissues, the speed of transmission depending upon the nature of the tissue. Provided the change in speed is great enough the sound waves will be reflected back to a detector. Bone and air stop all sound wave transmission, thus ultrasonography is principally used in the investigation of soft tissues.

Table A1.13 Sialography in salivary gland disease

Disorder	Sialographic appearance
Calculi	Dilatation of ducts distal to the calculus; if radio-opaque, the calculus will also be detected on the plain film taken before sialography
Strictures	Dilatation of ducts distal to the stricture; narrowing at stricture
Sjögren's syndrome Recurrent parotitis in adults	Dilatation of ducts and acini Pooling of contrast medium in the dilated regions give rise to a 'snow-storm' radiographic appearance, known as sialectasis; as disease progresses, so the areas of pooling increase in size and number
Neoplasia	
Benign	Displacement of the normal ductal network Slight retention of contrast medium within the gland after a sialogogue has been given
Malignant	Destruction of the ductal network Irregular pooling of contrast medium and retention after sialogogue
Extra-glandular masses	Displacement of the normal ductal network No retention of contrast medium after a sialogogue

A1.14   (a) The patient has a mild, skeletal class III, dental-base relationship (ANB—1.5°). The facial proportions and maxillary/mandibular plane angle are average (27°).

The upper and lower incisors are proclined (122° and 103° to the maxillary and mandibular planes, respectively) and would meet edge to edge but for the open bite.

(b) This radiograph shows all the characteristic features of an atypical (endogenous) tongue behaviour.

(i) Upper and lower incisors are proclined.
(ii) Open bite (8 mm) between the central incisors.
(iii) The overbite reduces markedly from canine to incisor regions.
(iv) In both arches the incisors lie well apical to the occlusal plane, producing a triangular inter-occlusal space.

Clinically, the patient had a marked lisp.

A1.15   (a) 1. Lateral wall of the orbit.
2. Lateral rectus muscle.
3. Optic nerve.
4. Posterior wall of the nasopharynx.

(b) Computerized tomography (CT) permits visualization of both soft and hard tissue lesions in areas usually inaccessible to conventional radiographic techniques. Hence in dentistry, CT has primarily been applied in the detection of fibrous dysplasia, maxillary cysts, and neoplasms of the maxillary and infra-temporal areas. However, the clinical application of CT is ever-widening and now includes the following.

(i) Antral disease:
Foreign bodies
Cysts
Neoplasms.

(ii) Skeletal disease:
     Osteomyelitis
     Osteoarthrosis (of temporomandibular joint)
     Rheumatoid arthritis (of temporomandibular joint)
     Primary neoplasms and metastases
     Fibrous dysplasia
     Paget's disease
     Cysts (e.g., keratocysts of mandible and maxilla)
     Sarcoidosis.

(iii) Other:
     Sjögren's syndrome
     Salivary neoplasms.

 Sialography may be combined with CT in the diagnosis of Sjögren's syndrome and salivary tumours.

PAPER 2 · QUESTIONS

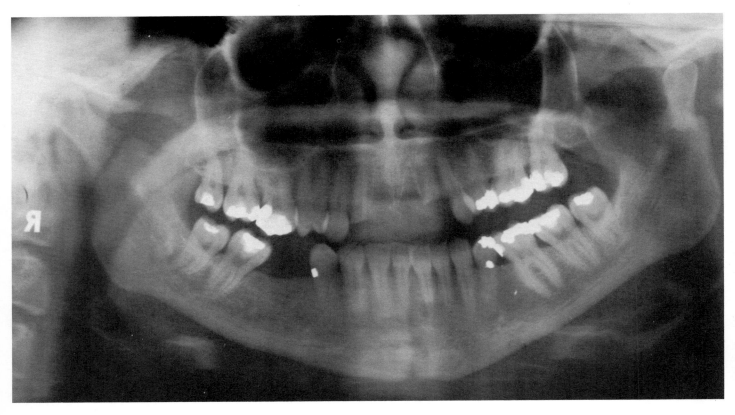

Q2.1   This patient was an allegedly innocent victim of an assault.
(a) Provide a diagnosis.
(b) What clinical feature often distinguishes a bilateral fracture of the mandibular condyles from a unilateral fracture?

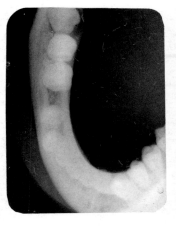
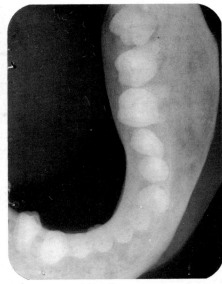

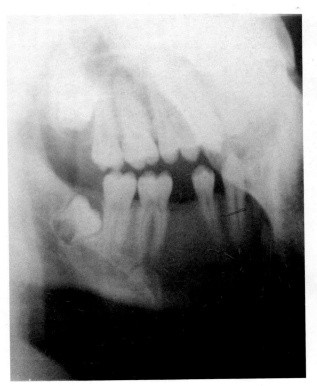
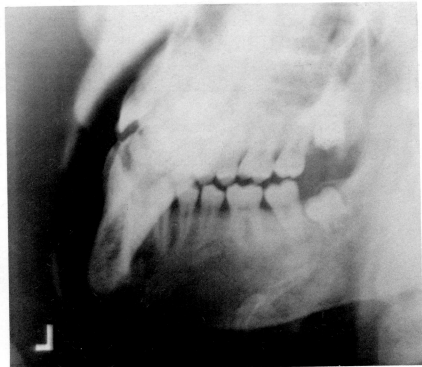

Q2.2   This 16 year old, medically fit male was referred by his dentist regarding an unusual radiographic appearance about ⌐67.

(a) Suggest a diagnosis.

(b) Routine serological investigations revealed:

total serum calcium 2.4 mmol/l
total serum phosphate 1.2 mmol/l
total serum alkaline phosphatase 10 KA units.

Are these results expected?

(c) What treatment is required?

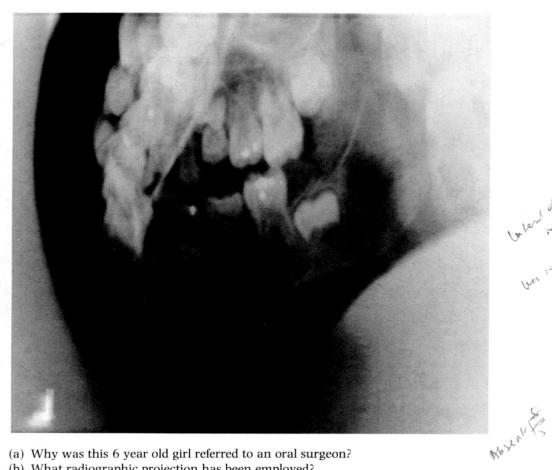

Q2.3   (a) Why was this 6 year old girl referred to an oral surgeon?
           (b) What radiographic projection has been employed?
           (c) What are the advantages of this technique compared with pantomography?

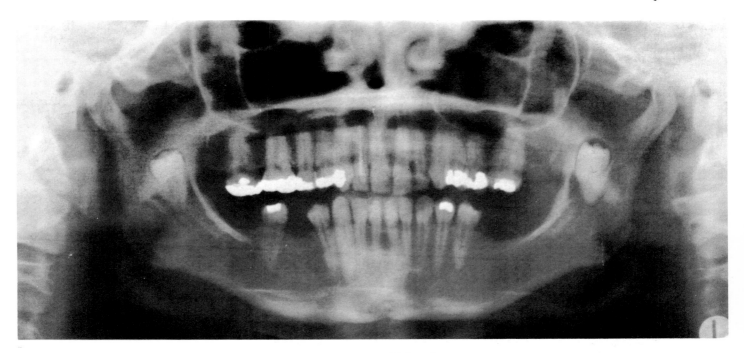

Q2.4   The patient is a 26 year old female.
(a) What treatment for the misplaced unerupted lower third molars would you advise?
(b) What would be the prognosis if the teeth were to be left in place?

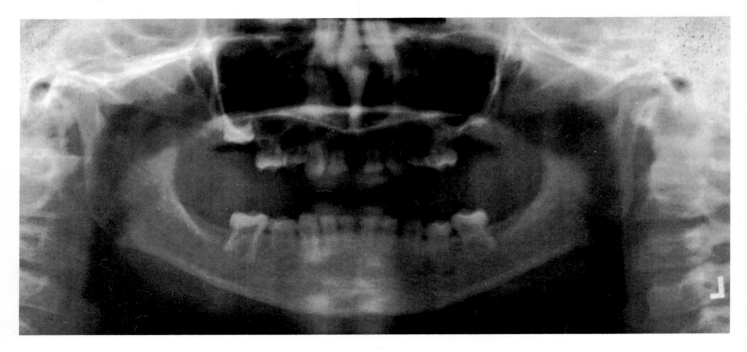

Q2.5   (a) What are the dental abnormalities of this 14 year old girl?
        (b) The patient has dry skin and a generalized lack of hair. Suggest a diagnosis.
        (c) What are the major clinical features of this disorder?

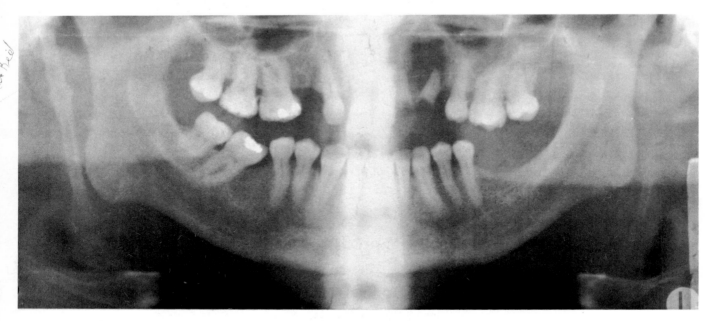

Q2.6   (a) What is the most likely diagnosis of the radiolucent area in the upper left jaw?
        (b) What other investigations would you do before operation?

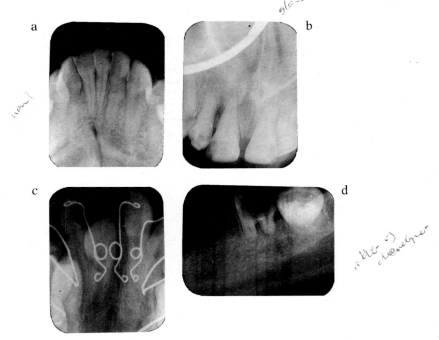

Q2.7   What are these film faults?

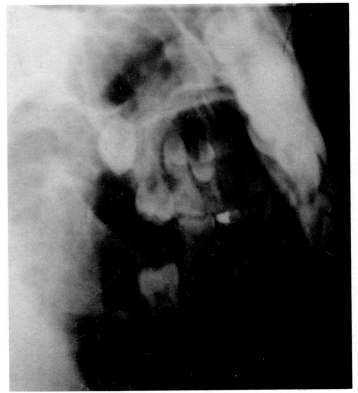

Q2.8   The X-ray report of this 7 year old patient suggested that no abnormalities were present.
(a) Why might the report be questioned?
(b) What is the appropriate management?

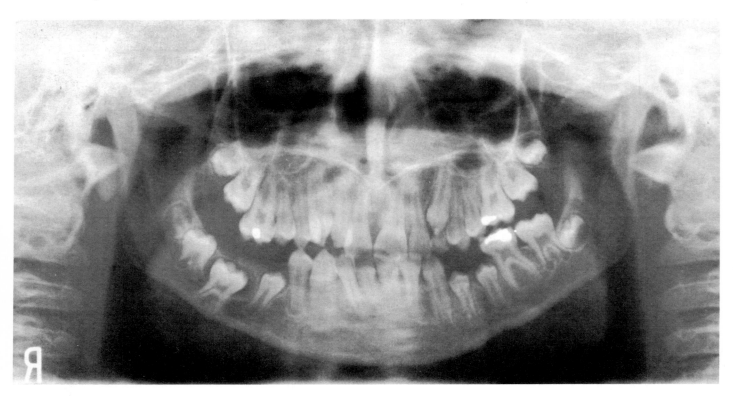

Q2.9   (a) Approximately how old is this patient?
             (b) Can the lower right first molar be expected to erupt?

11 – 12 y

PAPER 2 · QUESTIONS

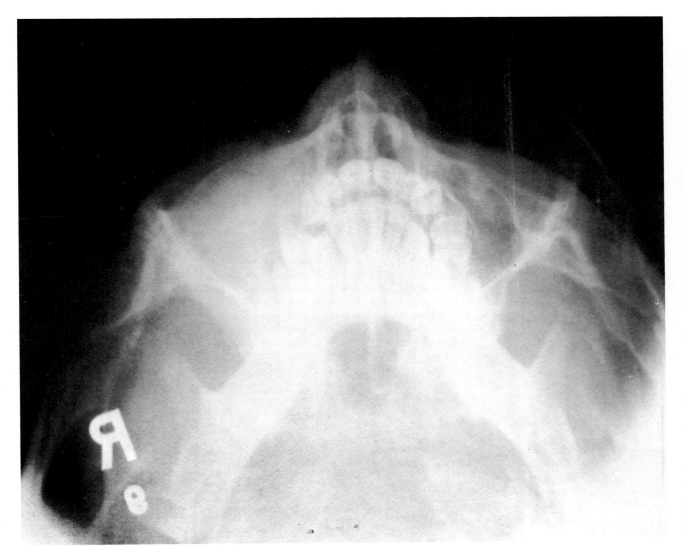

Q2.10   (a) What abnormalities are shown?

(b) What other investigations may help to clarify the nature and extent of this lesion?

(c) Why is this radiographic view particularly useful for investigating the middle third of the facial skeleton?

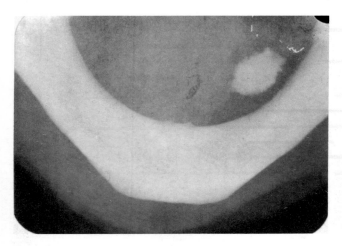

Q2.11   (a) What radiographic view is this?
              (b) How can you localize this radio-opacity?

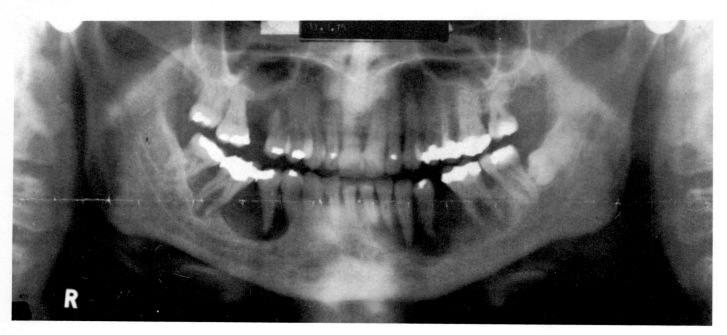

Q2.12   This patient is a medically fit 14 year old female.
              (a) What abnormalities are present? Suggest a diagnosis.
              (b) What immunological abnormality is implicated in the aetiology of this disorder?
              (c) How might you manage this patient?

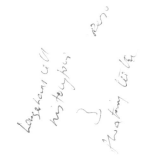

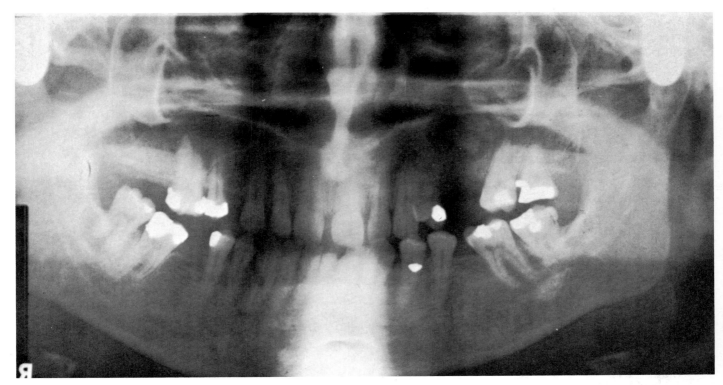

Q2.13   (a) What maxillary lesion(s) is shown here?
            (b) How can this problem be surgically managed?

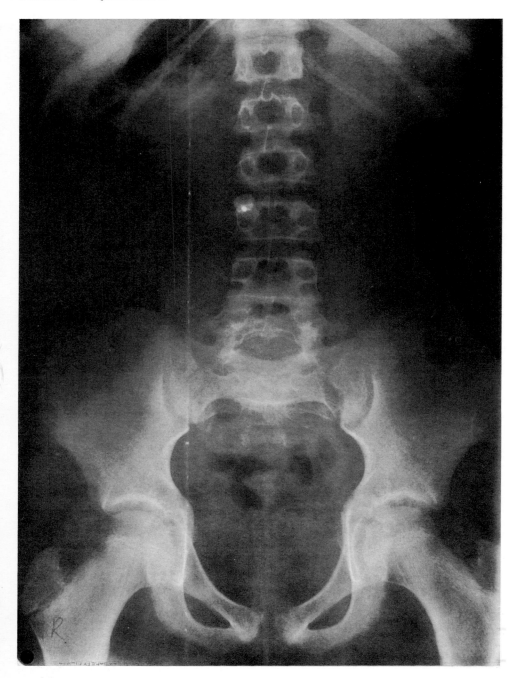

Q2.14   (a) What is the dentally relevant abnormality?
            (b) What is the prognosis?

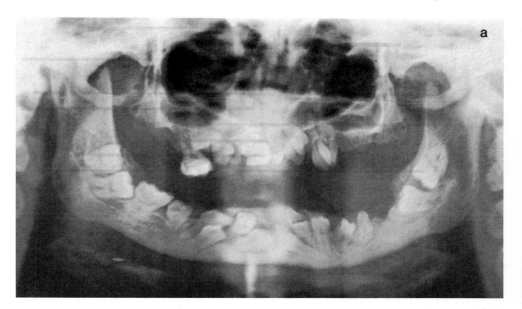

Cleidocranial dysostosis

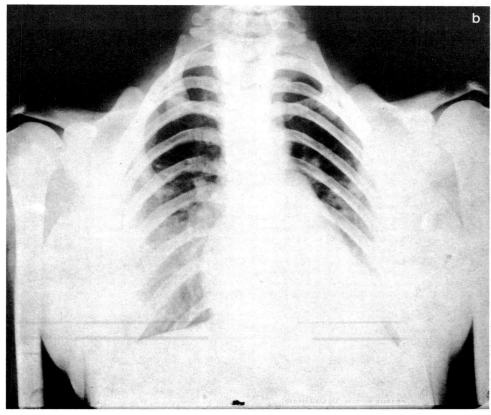

Q2.15   (a) What radiographic abnormalities are present in this film of a 14 year old girl?
        (b) Film (b) is of the same patient. What is the diagnosis, and what are the other
            orofacial features of this disorder?
        (c) List the systemic disorders in which delayed eruption of teeth may be a feature.

PAPER 2 · ANSWERS

A2.1 (a) There are fractures of the mandibular body (symphysis), and left and right necks of condyle. In addition 1|1 have recently been lost and there are fractures of the roots of 2|2.

(b) Bilateral fractures of the mandibular condyle can cause a downward and forward displacement of the mandibular body resulting in an anterior open bite and premature contact of the occlusal surfaces of the posterior teeth. Le Fort fractures in the middle third of the face can also cause such occlusal problems.

A2.2 (a) The bone has a typically 'ground-glass' or 'orange-peel' appearance. The young age of the patient and the unilateral nature of the lesion suggest fibrous dysplasia.

(b) Levels of serum calcium, phosphate, and alkaline phosphatase are all within normal limits—this *is* expected for fibrous dysplasia.

(c) Unless the patient has any notable facial asymmetry, no surgical treatment is required. The patient should, however, be reviewed to ensure no continued growth of the lesion.

A2.3 (a) Absent |$\frac{5}{5}$.

(b) Oblique lateral mandible projection.

(c) (i) No need for costly radiographic equipment—oblique lateral views can be obtained using a conventional dental X-ray unit (70 kV minimal).

(ii) Carious lesions and periodontal disease can be more readily detected on oblique lateral views than by pantomography.

(iii) Radiographs of wheelchair-bound patients cannot be obtained using an pantomogram, but oblique lateral views can be obtained with the patient sitting down.

(iv) Oblique laterals, result in less radiation than pantomography.

A2.4 (a) Although the patient is relatively young, she has no erupted lower molars and the $\overline{76|67}$ are absent, so she is reaching the point where a lower denture would be necessary. However, the unerupted, misplaced lower third molars are nowhere near the denture-bearing area and could safely be left in place. They are completely symptomless and would probably never have been noticed had the general practitioner not had a pantomography machine.

(b) It is common to find unerupted or misplaced third molars in otherwise edentulous mandibles. Occasionally a communication arises between the crown of the tooth and the mouth, which can lead to infection especially if the tooth is under the denture-bearing area. In middle to old age the outlines of the original follicle around the crown and the periodontal ligament space become indistinct and resorption of the surfaces of the crown and root can occur. Dentigerous cysts are also fairly commonly associated with unerupted third molars, but are more likely to develop in the early decades of life.

A.2.5 (a) Hypodontia. Severe attrition of anterior deciduous teeth.

(b) Hypohidrotic ectodermal dysplasia.

(c) Ectodermal dysplasia is often an X-linked recessive disorder clinically characterized by hypodontia, hypotrichosis (lack of normal amounts of hair), and hypohidrosis (reduced ability to sweat). There is an underlying developmental defect of ectodermal tissue.

Aside from hypodontia or anodontia of the deciduous and permanent teeth, other orofacial manifestations include lack of nasal bridge, frontal bossing, loss of vertical face height, protuberant lower lips, and prominent ears. The anterior teeth of affected patients, if present, may have a conical shape (Fig. A2.5).

Lack of sweat glands causes hypohidrosis and heat intolerance. The skin is dry, due to lack of sebaceous glands, and soft. There is a generalized lack of hair.

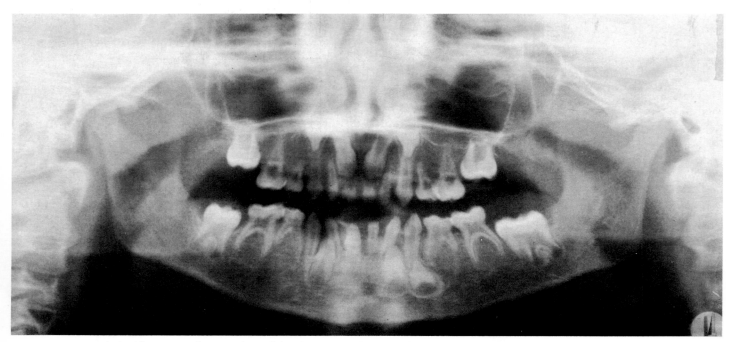

Fig. A2.5 This patient has ectodermal dysplasia: note the conical shape of the crowns of the anterior teeth.

A2.6 (a) Periodontal (dental, radicular, apical) cyst.

(b) A pantomograph is inadequate to show the full extent of a cyst such as this. A naso-occlusal view is useful to show the posterior extent and a postero-anterior view of the skull would show the proximity to the floor of the nose. Additional radiographic views are important, not only practically but also medico-legally.

In addition to vitality tests, periapical views of adjacent teeth may help in deciding whether they are involved. It would also be wise to do standard haematological investigations before any surgery because bleeding from this region can be profuse.

Incidentally, the right stylohyoid ligament is extensively calcified.

A2.7 (a) X-ray film damaged by nail of dark-room operator—this could be misinterpreted as a fracture!

(b) Patient still wearing metal-framed glasses.

(c) Patient still wearing orthodontic appliance.

(d) Film damage from roller of developer.

A2.8 (a) The radiologist has missed absence of $\overline{5|}$; failed eruption of $\overline{6|}$, possibly as a result of ankylosis; absence of $\overline{7|}$.

(b) Surgical removal of $\overline{6|}$.

Other procedures such as transplantation or exposure and orthodontic alignment are either unlikely to be successful or impossible.

Simply leaving $\overline{6|}$ is also unwise as resorption of $\overline{E|}$ and/or dentigerous cyst formation is possible.

A2.9 (a) The patient is about 11 to 12 years of age.

(b) Eruption of $\overline{6|}$ is unlikely because this tooth has formed roots and may be ankylosed. After apical closure all teeth are less likely to erupt even when surgically uncovered. Lower first molars in particular have an extremely poor prognosis for so doing; many appear to be ankylosed and fail to erupt even when orthodontic traction is applied.

A2.10 (a) This occipito-mental radiograph shows uniform radio-opacity of the right maxillary antrum. While the lateral antral wall appears normal, the antero-superior aspect demonstrates expansion and loss of cortical outline in the region of the infra-orbital margin. Compared with the contralateral side there is loss of trabeculation over the right antrum. The appearance of the right maxillary antrum is consistent with a diagnosis of fibrous dysplasia as the area has a 'ground glass' appearance.

(b) Radiographic findings point to a diagnosis of a fibro-osseous lesion, though it is important to rule out neoplasia. Incisional biopsy via a Caldwell–Luc approach under local analgesia should therefore be carried out.

Fibro-osseous lesions principally comprise fibrous dysplasia, Paget's disease, and giant-cell disorders. Blood and urinary chemistry can help in differential diagnosis (Table A2.10). In this case, the unifocal nature of the condition was confirmed by radionuclide scanning (Fig. A2.10a). This scan of the right face demonstrates

Table A2.10 Serum biochemical anomalies in fibro-osseous lesions

	Serum calcium (*total* calcium† 2.3–2.6 mmol/l)	Serum phosphate† (0.8–1.5 mmol/l)	Serum alkaline phosphatase† (30–110 iu/l; 3–13 KA units)
Fibrous dysplasia*	N	N	N or ↑
Cherubism*	N	N	N or ↑
Paget's disease*	N	N	↑
Primary hyperparathyroidism:			
without bone lesions	↑	↓	N
with bone lesions	↑	N or ↓	↑
Secondary hyperparathyroidism:			
	N or ↓	N or ↓	N or ↑
Tertiary hyperparathyroidism:			
without bone lesions	↑	N or ↓	N or ↑
with bone lesions	↑	N or ↓	N

N = Normal.

*Urinary hydroxyproline may also be raised, particularly in Paget's disease.

†Levels vary with each reference group.

obvious increased uptake or a 'hot spot' affecting the maxilla. There is no obvious increased uptake in any other part of the facial skeleton. The appearance of the condylar region is within normal limits—the area of increased technetium uptake reflects increased activity in this growth area.

Computerized (axial) tomography (Fig. A2.10b) demonstrates the extent of the lesion. Interestingly, there is aeration of the medial aspect of the antrum not readily apparent on the occipito-mental radiograph. The scan shows slight anterior expansion of the facial skeleton, but no real posterior extension. Computerized tomography is particularly useful in assessing the posterior extension of antral lesions.

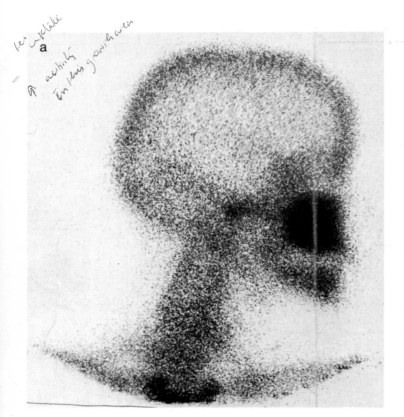
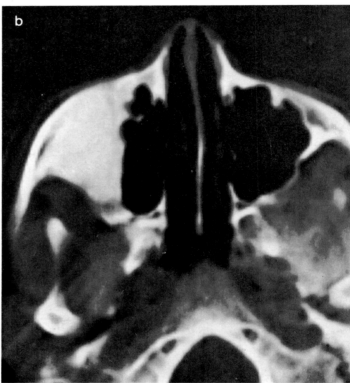

Fig. A2.10 (a) There is accumulation of radionucleotide in the area of the right maxilla.
(b) Computed tomography reveals a solid lesion in the right maxillary antrum.

(c) The occipitomental view is particularly useful for examining the middle part of the facial skeleton, principally because the structures of the cranial base are not superimposed. Whilst the X-ray beam passes through the cranial base and the cranial vault, it does so at right angles and parallel to the principal buttresses within the facial skeleton. The latter structures are therefore particularly clear.

A convenient way of assessing an occipito-mental view is to identify a series of arcs, starting with the cranial vault and working inferiorly. Thus, after examination of the cranium, the supra-orbital ridges and frontal sinus are next examined. The next arc comprises the zygomatic arches, body of zygoma, infra-orbital margins, and nasal bones. Following this the coronoid process, lateral antral wall, antra, and inferior nasal skeleton are identified. Though more inferior parts of the facial skeleton are included in occipito-mental films, these are usually not as clearly defined. Lower arcs may include the upper alveolus, lower alveolus, and lower border of the mandible.

A2.11   (a) Lower occlusal view of anterior floor of mouth and the anterior lower area of the mandible. A submandibular salivary calculus is present in association with the left submandibular gland and/or duct.

            (b) (i) Clinical examination: inspection and palpation of the floor of mouth. The patient should tip his or her head forwards; this ensures the muscles of the floor of the mouth are relaxed, making tactile examination much easier.

                 (ii) Radiographic examination: to determine accurately the vertical position of the radio-opacity a second radiograph taken in a second plane should be obtained, e.g., a pantomograph or oblique lateral. However, in this particular instance, palpation easily allowed localization of the lesion.

A2.12   (a) (i) Gross loss of periodontal bone about $\overline{8754\,|\,346}$.

                 (ii) Absence of $\dfrac{6\,|\,8}{6\,|\,5}$.

                 (iii) Horizontal impaction of $\overline{8}$.

                 (iv) There is also a root filling in $\underline{5}$.

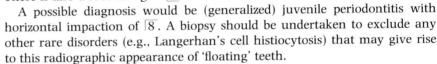

                     A possible diagnosis would be (generalized) juvenile periodontitis with horizontal impaction of $\overline{8}$. A biopsy should be undertaken to exclude any other rare disorders (e.g., Langerhan's cell histiocytosis) that may give rise to this radiographic appearance of 'floating' teeth.

            (b) Reduced neutrophil chemotaxis.

            (c) (i) This radiograph does not reveal any details about the condition of the periodontal bone about all the upper teeth, thus periapicals should be taken.

                 (ii) As the prognosis of $\overline{75\,|\,346}$ is so poor, they should be extracted.

                 (iii) Improvement of oral hygiene.

                 (iv) Systemic tetracyclines may be needed if there is severe acute inflammation of periodontal pockets.

                 (v) Periodontal surgery to eliminate deep pockets.

                 (vi) Routine patient recall to ensure maintenance of good oral hygiene.

                 (vii) Surgical removal of $\underline{8}$ is indicated because this is probably in communication with the mouth.

A2.13   (a) There is a root and cyst associated with the left maxillary antrum.

            (b) The root (and cyst) should be removed under general anaesthesia, the approach being via the buccal aspect of the extraction socket. Alternatively a Caldwell–Luc procedure might be undertaken in which the approach is via the upper left canine fossa.

A2.14   (a) There is a crown of a tooth in the gastro-intestinal tract. The patient swallowed it after being assaulted.

            (a) It will most likely pass uneventfully.

If a foreign object passes into an unprotected pharynx, the dental procedure must be stopped and the patient should try and cough out the object. The patient must not be slapped on the back, this merely sends the object further down into the respiratory tract. If the object cannot be dislodged, the Heimlich manœuvre should be attempted (Fig. A2.14). If this fails, the patient should be immediately referred to a local Accident and Emergency department for chest and abdominal radiographs, and endoscopy.

     Prevention is the best treatment—thus all dental procedures that might cause objects or material to pass into the pharynx should be undertaken using rubber dam or with the patient in an upright position, or the pharynx should be protected with a piece of gauze placed between the dorsum of tongue and palate. It is also useful to use a parachute chain or to tie floss around endodontic instruments.

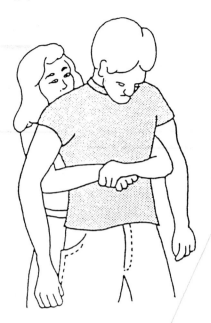

Fig. A2.14 The Heimlich manœuvre. The operator grasps one fist with the opposite hand and presses the abdominal cavity inwards and upwards (Courtesy of British Dental Journal).

A2.15 (a) (i) Delayed eruption of all permanent teeth apart from 6⌋.
  (ii) Multiple supernumerary teeth, especially in upper incisor region.
  (iii) Absence of all upper molars other than 6⌋.
  (iv) Multiple impacted teeth.
  (v) Short, thinned tooth roots.

(b) Cleidocranial dysplasia (dysostosis): the radiograph shows clavicular hypoplasia.
  (i) Delayed closure of fontanelles.
  (ii) Delayed fusion of cranial sutures.
  (iii) Multiple wormian bones of cranium (Fig. A2.15).
  (iv) Prominent parietal, frontal, and occipital bones.
  (v) Narrow, high-arched palate.
  (vi) Maxillary hypoplasia.
  (vii) Retention of deciduous teeth.
  (viii) Increased frequency of dentigerous cysts.
  (ix) Roots of teeth may be short, thin, and deformed.

(c) Aside from cleidocranial dysplasia, delayed eruption of teeth can occur in hypoparathyroidism, hypopituitarism, hypothyroidism, Down's syndrome, and osteopetrosis. It can also be a complication of malnutrition, irradiation of the head and neck, cytotoxic therapy, and several rare genetic disorders.

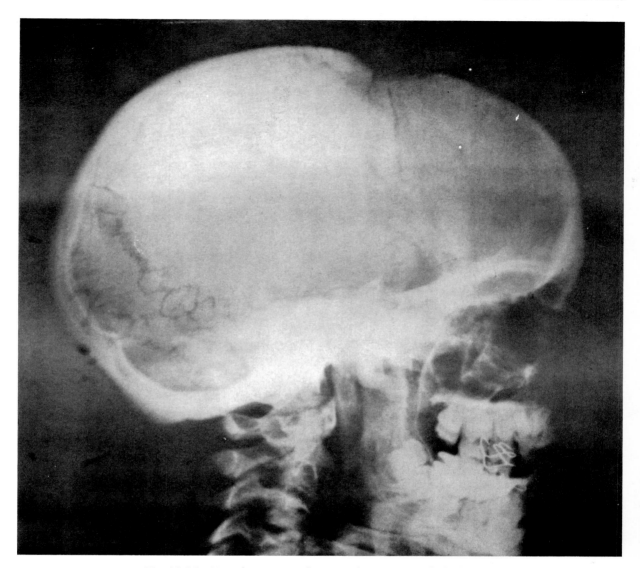

Fig. A2.15   Note the wormian bones in this patient with cleidocranial dysplasia.

PAPER 3 · QUESTIONS

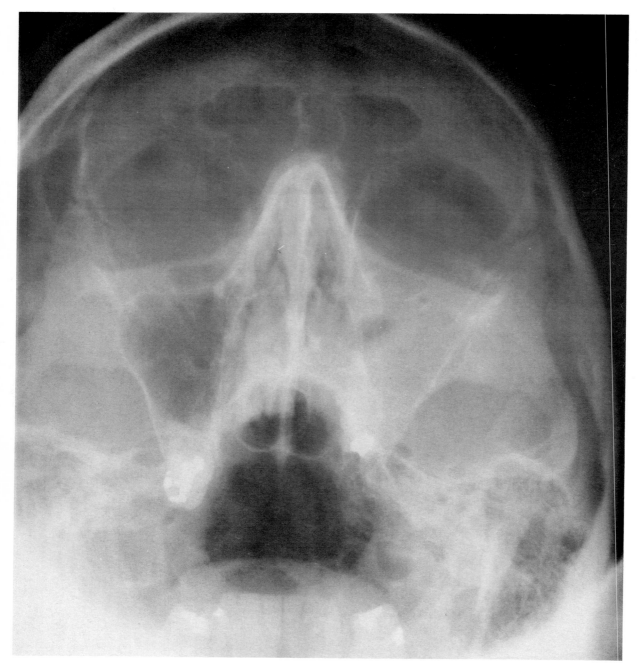

Q3.1 This patient is a medically fit 40 year old male referred to an oral surgeon for closure of an oro-antral fistula in the ⌊6 area.
(a) Provide a diagnosis.
(b) Conservative measures failed to eradicate any of the radiographic features—what surgical treatment is required?

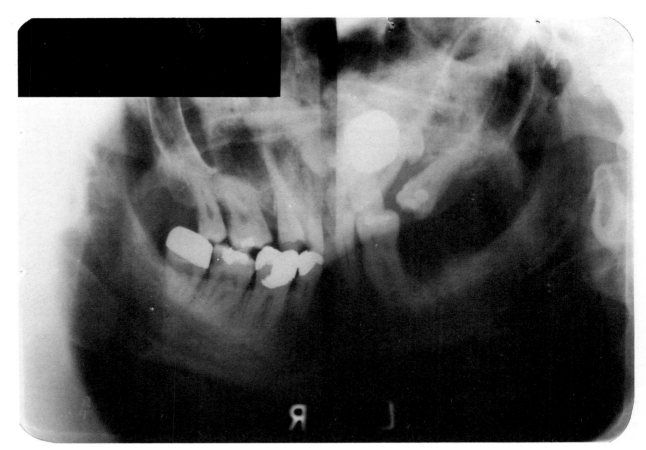

Q3.2   (a) What problems are present in this patient?
(b) What radiographic projection is this?
(c) What are the advantages of this projection when compared with intra-oral projections?

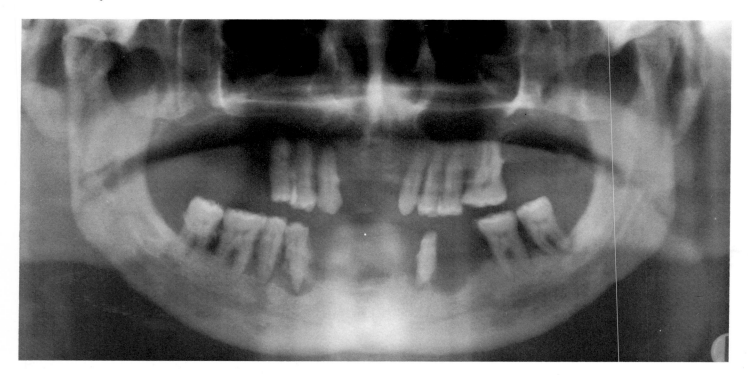

Q3.3 This is a 40 year old patient with Down's syndrome.
(a) What is the likely cause of this patient's periodontal problem?
(b) What orofacial anomalies can arise in Down's syndrome?

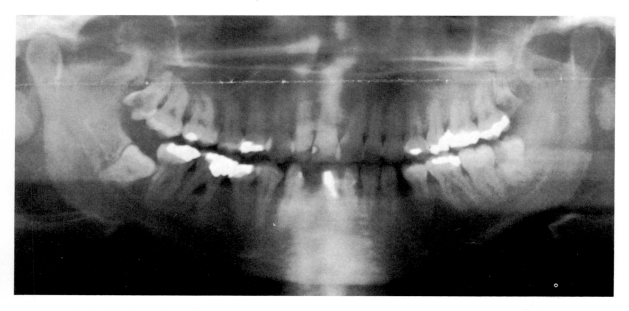

Q3.4 (a) Which teeth would you remove from this patient?
(b) The patient is allergic to penicillin and has a prosthetic mitral valve. What additional precautions are required therefore when removing this patient's teeth?

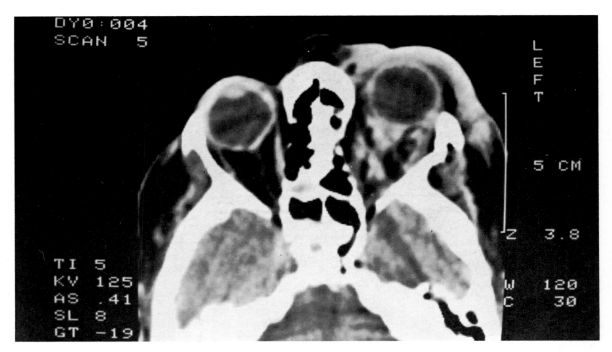

```
DY0:004
SCAN    5

                                    L
                                    E
                                    F
                                    T

                                  .5 CM

                                Z   3.8

TI  5
KV  125
AS  .41                          W   120
SL  8                            C    30
GT  -19
```

Q3.5   This 30 year old woman was involved in a road traffic accident and sustained trauma
to the left side of the face and head resulting in unconsciousness.
(a) What bony injuries are apparent?
(b) What has been the effect of the injury, on the left eye?

proptosis

*depressed frontal #
enlr pyros n S. hel
                margin*

damage to (L) ethmoid

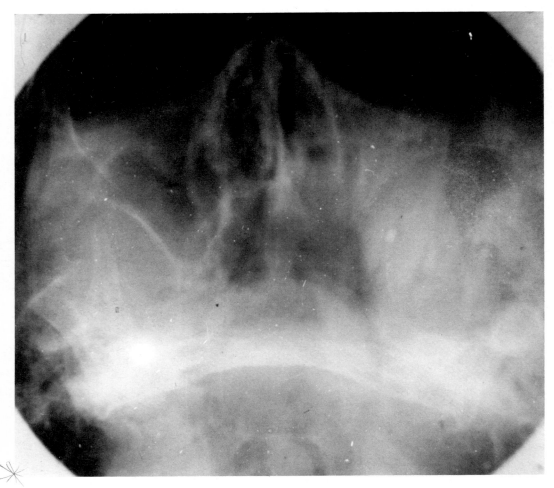

Q3.6   This 69 year old patient attended his dentist complaining of a lump on the upper left side of his palate.
(a) Suggest the likely diagnosis.
(b) What additional radiological investigations will help precisely delineate this lesion?
(c) What are the clinical features of this disorder?

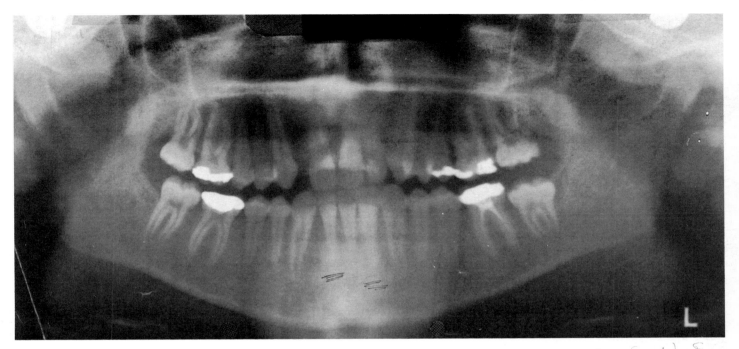

Q3.7 The patient is 28 years of age. Which teeth are missing?

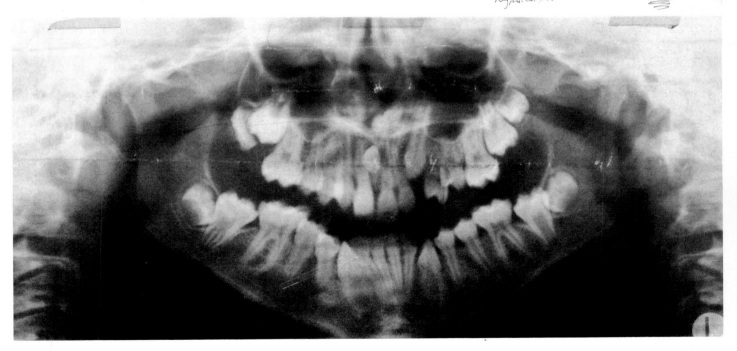

Q3.8 (a) What is overlying the occlusal surface of 7|?
(b) What is the abnormal structure in the maxillary midline?
(c) What, if any, are the orthodontic problems?

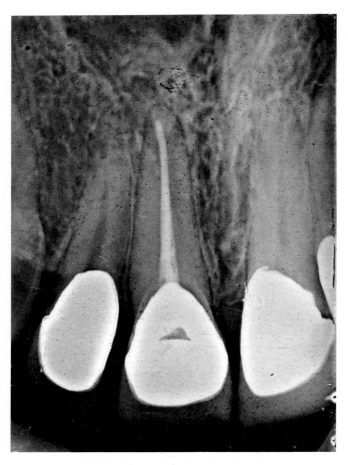

Q3.9 (a) What radiographic technique does this illustrate?
(b) List the possible advantages and disadvantages of this technique.

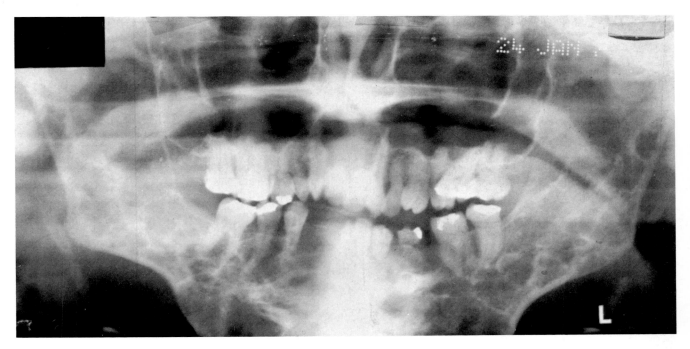

Q3.10 In childhood this patient had an unusually chubby face.
(a) What is the diagnosis?
(b) What is the treatment of this disorder?

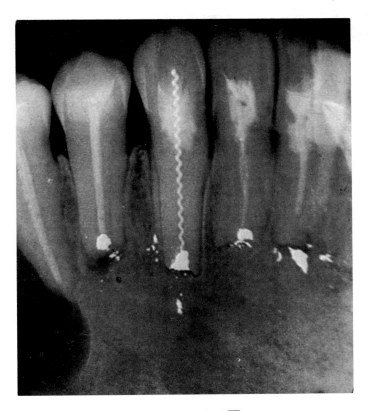

Q3.11 (a) What is the radio-opacity in the root canal of $\overline{3}|$?
(b) What are the main indications for apicectomy and retrograde root filling of teeth?
(c) What types of mucoperiosteal flap can be used for apicectomies?

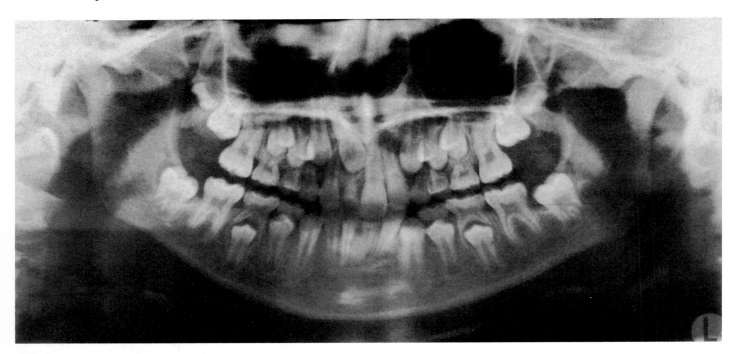

Q3.12   What is the cause of the unerupted right maxillary central incisor in this 12 year old patient?

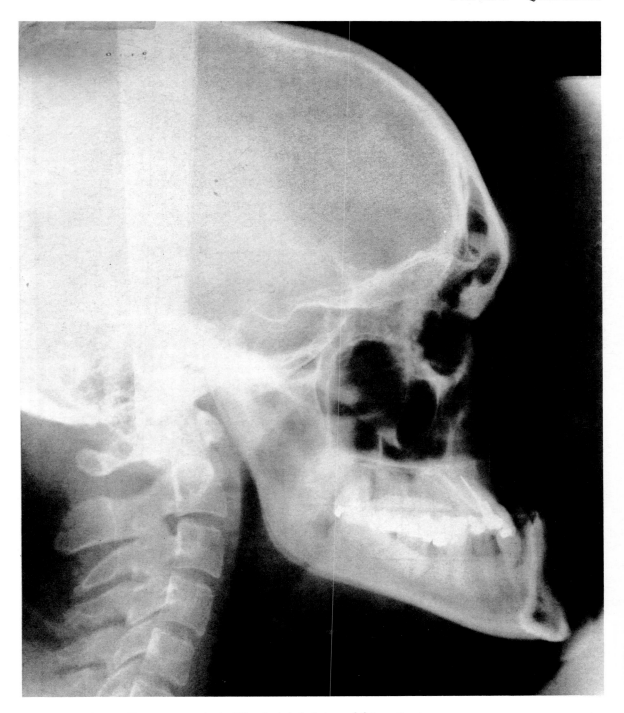

Q3.13   Give an appraisal of the facial skeleton of this patient.

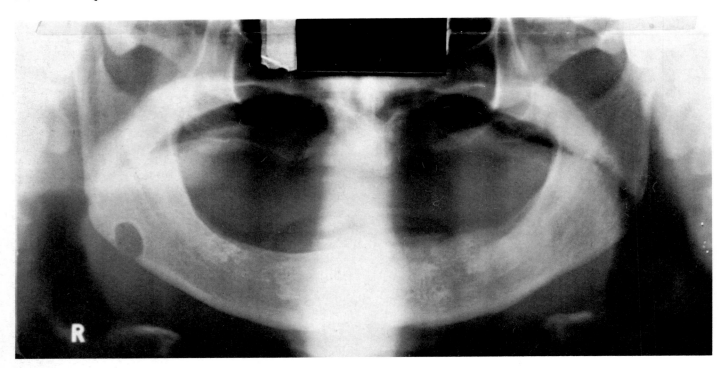

Q3.14   This patient had a root removed from $\overline{8|}$ region one year before this pantomograph was taken.
(a) What is the lesion?
(b) What is the origin of the lesion?

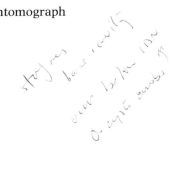

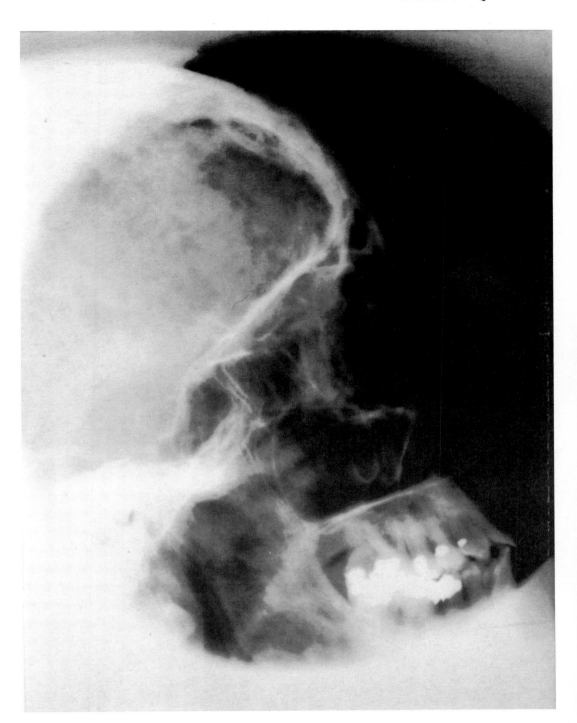

Q3.15   (a) This patient complained of generalized bone pain and had a raised plasma viscosity with serum IgG paraproteins. What is the diagnosis?
(b) What are the common biochemical markers of this disorder?
(c) What are the oral manifestations of this disorder?

PAPER 3 · ANSWERS

A3.1   (a) The left maxillary antrum has a uniform radio-opaque appearance. There is no disruption of the bony margins of the sinus, thus neoplasia or dysplasia seems unlikely. The probable diagnosis is chronic sinusitis.

(b) Surgical closure of the fistula and intranasal antrostomy—this latter procedure ensures efficient drainage by creating an opening in the medial wall of the sinus at the level of the nasal floor. In addition, the lining of a chronically inflamed sinus usually has a large number of oedematous polyps that can be removed before the fistula is closed.

A3.2   (a) (i) Recurrent caries in $\overline{876|}$ and possibly $\overline{5|}$.

(ii) Tilted $|8$.

(iii) Periodontal bone loss about all standing molars.

(iv) Submerged $|\underline{E}$.

(b) Rotated lateral mandible ('bimolar') projection although the left projection is rather oblique.

(c) (i) Low radiation exposure.

(ii) The bimolar projection is simple, rapid, and not intra-oral. It is thus highly suitable for the radiographic investigation of children, handicapped patients, and individuals with a profound gagging reflex.

A3.3   (a) Poor oral hygiene maintenance. This is suggested by the heavy deposits of calculus about all remaining teeth.

Patients with Down's syndrome can have a number of subtle immunodeficiencies that may (although it remains to be proven) accentuate periodontal destruction. Possibly the most important immune defect of Down's syndrome that will increase susceptibility to periodontal disease is reduced neutrophil function.

(b) Craniofacial anomalies include:

Brachycephaly
Flattened occiput
✗ Late closure of fontanelles
Shortened antero-posterior skull diameter
Short neck (and dislocation of atlas)
Hypoplastic or absent sinuses
Mid-face hypoplasia
Class III skeletal profile
Low-set, malformed ears
Sparse eyebrows
Recurrent ocular and upper respiratory tract infections.

Oral anomalies include:

Thickened, everted lips
Relative macroglossia
Tongue protrusion
Open mouth posture
Palatal abnormalities
Delayed eruption of decidious and permanent dentitions
Oligodontia
Crown abnormalities (e.g., bulbous or conical crowns)
Short roots
Enamel hypoplasia
Increased susceptibility to periodontal disease.

A3.4   (a) Both upper third molars are grossly carious and need removal. $\overline{6|}$ has extensive periodontal bone loss below the bifurcation and there are periapical radiolucent areas around both roots. $\overline{8|}$ is also grossly carious, and deserves a high priority for removal because:

          (i)   there is a strong possibility of pulpitis leading to periapical periodontitis;

          (ii) a vertically impacted lower third molar with at least three curved roots is more difficult to remove in an emergency than any of the other carious teeth.

          $\overline{8|}$ is symptomless, well enclosed within bone, and furthermore has roots closely associated with the mandibular canal. It could be safely left in place.

     (b) Patients with prosthetic heart valves are almost always receiving anticoagulant therapy, thus before treatment the international normalized ratio (INR) must be checked and warfarin therapy altered to ensure an INR of below 2 on the day of oral surgery.

          Antiobiotic cover is essential: the patient belongs to the high-risk category for endocarditis and, as the patient is allergic to penicillin, the cover required is pre-operative 1 g vancomycin given intravenously over 60 minutes followed by 120 mg gentamicin, intravenously.

A3.5   (a) There is a large depressed frontal fracture also involving the supra-orbital margin. There is also damage to the left ethmoid.

     (b) The left eye shows proptosis and there is evidence of damage and bleeding around the musculature and optic nerve of this eye. The right eye shows clearly its extra-ocular muscles and optic nerve. Normal vision was retained in the left eye, although initially there was double vision due to displacement of the eye. Vision returned to normal after the bony injury was treated with combined neuro-surgery/maxillo-facial surgery.

A3.6   (a) There is a large radio-opacity in the left maxillary region. The radio-opacity has poorly defined margins and has caused destruction of the lateral margin of the maxillary sinus. There is also involvement of the infra-orbital margin. The lesion is less radiodense than bone but is of uniform radiodensity.

          The most likely diagnosis is a carcinoma of the left maxillary antrum.

     (b) Computed tomography (CT) or magnetic resonance imaging (MRI).

     (c) Clinical features of carcinoma of the maxillary sinus may include:

          Pain
          Palatal swelling, which may ulcerate
          Loosening and mobility of upper teeth
          Paraesthesia/anaesthesia in distribution of the maxillary nerve
          Swelling over cheek
          Epistaxis
          Epiphora
          Proptosis
          Cervical lymphadenopathy.

A3.7   All four third molars, $2|$ and one of the lower incisors are absent. This is a patient with hypodontia.

A3.8   (a) The image of $7|$ has the partially formed crown of the third molar superimposed upon it. There is seldom any need for intervention in such a case as the third molar is usually buccal to the crown of the second molar. The second molar usually erupts without any difficulty but progress of such cases should be carefully monitored.

(b) There is a midline supernumerary tooth (inverted mesiodens) lying between the roots of the upper central incisors. 2|, although present, is palatally misplaced and superimposed on the image of 1|.

(c) There is generalized crowding in both arches, demonstrated by a shortage of space for the canines in both arches and the presence of upper molar 'stacking'. In the lower arch, crowding at the back of the arch is expressed by mild impaction of second molars, which are also overlapped by the third molar tooth germs.

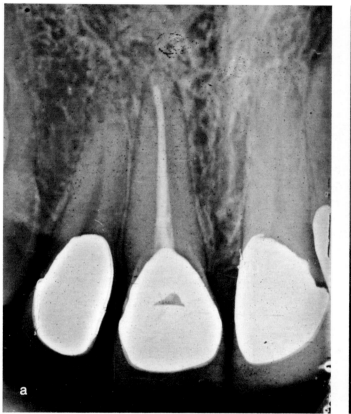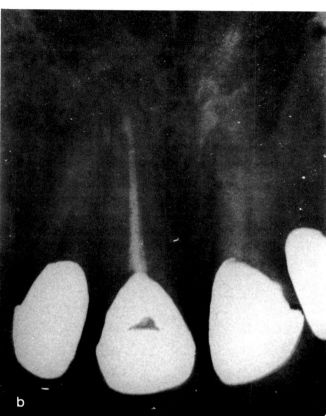

Fig. A3.9 This comparison of xeroradiography (a) and conventional radiography (b) illustrates the higher definition that can be obtained by xeroradiography.

A3.9   Xeroradiography

(a) Xeroradiography is a radiographic technique in which X-ray images are initially captured on a photoconductive plate and then transferred onto adhesive tape (c.f. photocopying). The major advantages of this technique are its ability to delineate clearly small structures and show areas of subtle density variation (Fig. A3.9).

Xeroradiography has occasionally been used in the investigation of some extra-oral lesions but the recent advances in computed tomography and magnetic resonance imaging (MRI) have superseded xeroradiography. Similarly, it was extensively used in mammography but has been succeedeed by newer techniques employing lower radiation doses.

(b) Advantages

(i) Reduced radiation exposure compared with conventional radiography.

(ii) Good imaging of small structures (e.g., bony trabeculae) and areas with subtle density differences, for example, localization of radiolucent or radio-opaque foreign bodies in soft tissues.

(iii) Images can be processed in a short time (less than 20 s). No wet processing, therefore no need for dark-room facilities.

Disadvantages

(i) New ultra-fast radiographic film now allows lower radiation doses.

(ii) Compared with conventional radiography using ultra-fast film, xero-radiography provides little additional clinical information in the assessment of carious lesions.

(iii) Non-availability and high capital costs and maintenance of suitable xero-radiographic equipment.

A3.10 (a) This is cherubism.

(b) Excess tissue may be excised but surgery should not be undertaken until the patient has reached puberty because only at this stage can the degree of facial deformity be anywhere near accurately estimated.

Cherubism is an autosomal dominant disorder in which males are twice as frequently affected as females. It is clinically characterized by multiple swellings of the jaws appearing at about 2 to 4 years of age, and then rapid and abnormal growth until about 7 years of age when disease progression slows or stops. All abnormal growth stops by puberty. The mandible is always affected, the maxilla is less frequently involved. There is usually bilateral involvement of the affected bones.

Facial deformity is the major clinical abnormality. Patients typically have a round, full face with prominent cheeks and jaws. Maxillary overgrowth causes upward displacement of the eyes and stretching of the skin below the eyes, thus exposing a rim of sclera below the iris. These features are said to give patients a cherubic appearance.

Reactive hyperplasia of submandibular lymph nodes contributes to the rounded facial appearance.

Dental anomalies include early exfoliation of deciduous teeth, and maldevelopment and delayed or failed eruption of permanent teeth.

Blood chemistry is usually normal but levels of serum alkaline phosphatase can be slightly raised during the osteolytic phase.

A3.11 (a) A spiral root-canal filler.

The filler became impacted within the canal preventing conventional orthograde root-canal filling, which is why apicectomy and retrograde root filling were undertaken.

(b) Apicectomy and retrograde root canal therapy are undertaken when there is periapical disease that does not resolve following orthograde root-canal therapy or when the latter is not possible, for example, with:

Post-crowned teeth
Large periapical granulomas or radicular cysts
Lateral perforation of root canal (e.g., ill-placed post-crown)
Fracture of root canal
Denticle (pulp stone)
Aberrant root-canal anatomy
Broken instrument in root canal
Failed removal of root-canal filling (e.g., apically placed silver points).

(c) Full buccal flaps are most frequently used although a flap formed by a semilunar incision 2 mm away from the gingival margin is occasionally employed.

A3.12 The unerupted central incisor in this 12 year old patient is either:
   (i) obstructed by a midline supernumerary tooth (mesiodens) or
   (ii) has been displaced and dilacerated by indirect violence transmitted through the deciduous incisor.

The weight of evidence is for a supernumerary tooth being the cause. There is no sign of dilaceration and even where the deciduous central incisor is retained following an injury severe enough to damage the underlying permanent incisor, it will seldom be retained to the age of 12 years as in this case. Closer inspection reveals the follicle of a supernumerary below the incisal edge of the unerupted tooth, although the supernumerary itself is obscured by the radio-opacity of the right central incisor crown. Periapical or naso-occlusal radiographs are better than pantomograms for examining the anterior region.

A3.13 The patient has a gross skeletal class III dental-base relationship with an ANB angle of $-15°$. This discrepancy is due both to a true mandibular protrusion (SNB = 99.5°) and a slight maxillary retrusion (SNA = 84.5°). The lower face height as a proportion of the total face height is slightly reduced (51 per cent) as is the maxillary/mandibular plane angle (16°). These features and the form of the mandible are strongly indicative of forward rotation of the mandible during growth.

As is often found in skeletal III-based, Class III malocclusions, the lower incisors are retroclined and the upper incisors proclined (128° and 77° to the maxillary and mandibular planes, respectively). There is a reversed overjet of 8 mm, and the overbite is increased at 10 mm.

A3.14 (a) This is a Stafne bone cavity (lingual mandibular bone cavity; Stafne cavity; latent bone cyst). These lesions characteristically occur *below* the inferior dental canal as here. Odontogenic cysts usually occur *above* the canal.

   (b) Submandibular salivary gland within bony tissue. These cavities are thought to arise from localized atrophy due to salivary gland tissue pressing on the lingual aspect of the mandibular body or angle.

A3.15 (a) Multiple myeloma—with widespread osteolytic lesions of the skull.

   (b) IgG (and occasionally IgA or IgM) paraproteins in the serum, and urinary Bence-Jones proteins, are the main biochemical markers of multiple myeloma.
       Other accompanying biochemical and haematological changes include plasmacytosis, normochromic normocytic anaemia, leukopenia, thrombocytopenia, elevated erythrocyte sedimentation rate (ESR) and plasma viscosity, and raised serum calcium levels. Serum uric acid can also be raised.

   (c) Osteolytic lesions of the jaws
       Root resorption and increased mobility of teeth
       Facial paraesthesia and anaesthesia due to myeloid deposits in maxilla and mandible
       Increased susceptibility to viral infections (particularly herpes simplex or zoster)
       Oral petechiae
       Gingival bleeding
       Pathological jaw fractures.

       If there is accompanying amyloidosis, oral deposits of amyloid, and purpura, may be seen.

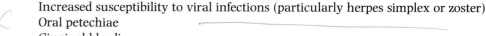

PAPER 4 · QUESTIONS

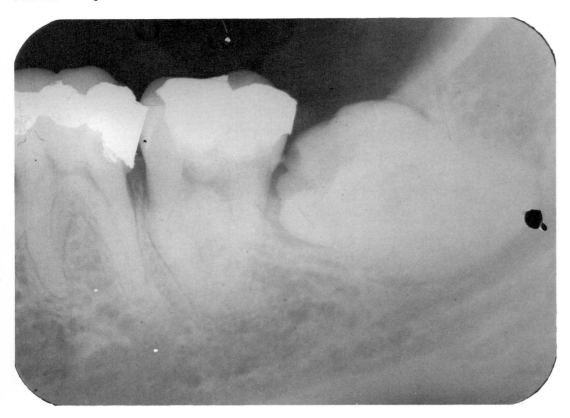

Q4.1   (a) Provide a diagnosis of the above patient's problem(s).

(b) What features allow accurate assessment of impacted lower third molars using periapical radiographs?

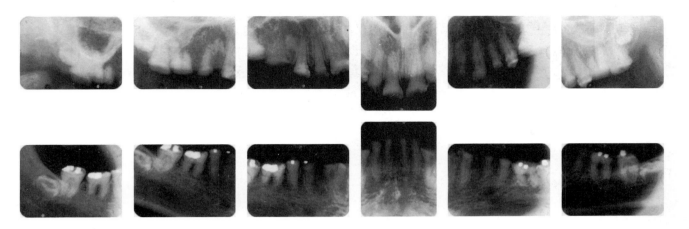

Q4.2   (a) This child has heavily discoloured teeth—why?

(b) The inheritance pattern of this condition is shown below. What is the mode of inheritance?

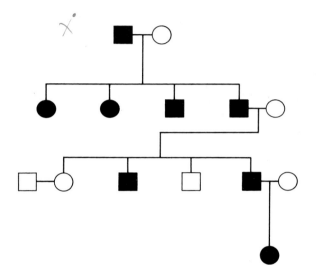

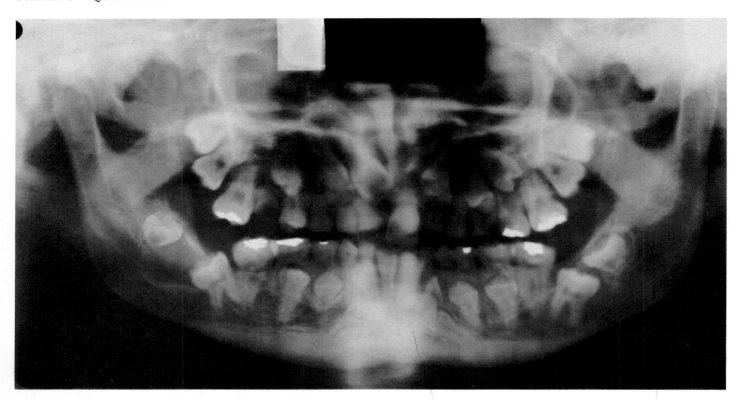

Q4.3   This is the radiograph of a 19 year old male with cleidocranial dysplasia. What dental anomalies are evident?

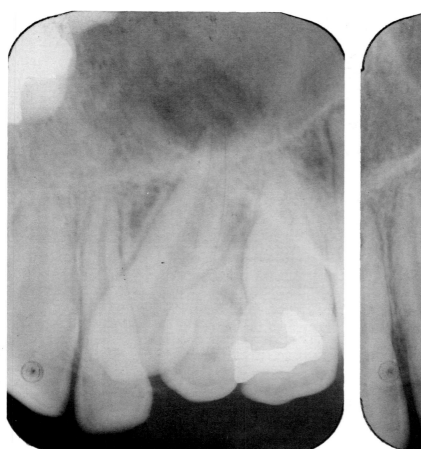
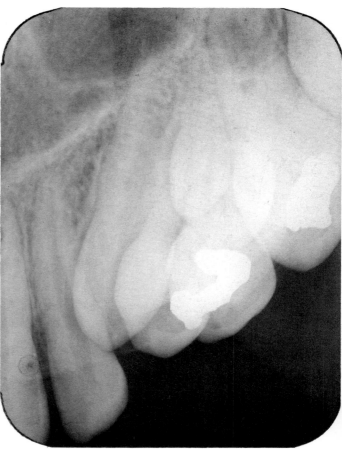

Q4.4   (a) This is an example of which radiographic technique?
         (b) Is the canine buccal or palatal to the dental arch?

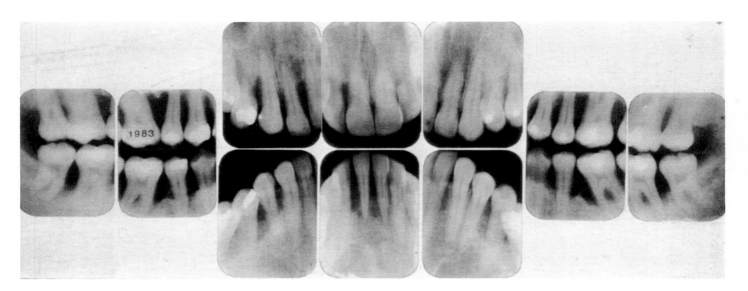

Q4.5   This is an apparently medically fit 31 year old female.
         (a) What abnormalities are present?
         (b) Which systemic disorders might account for this problem?

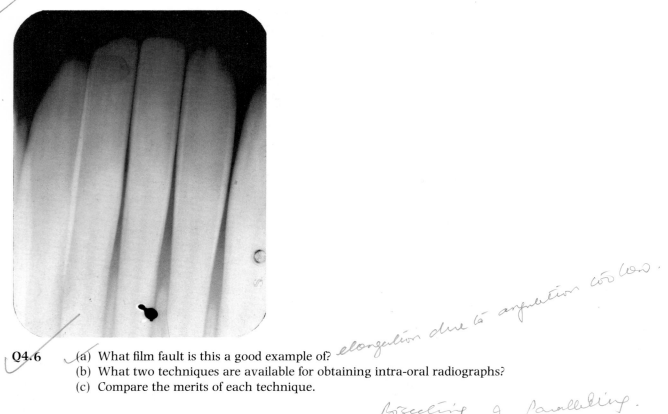

Q4.6   (a) What film fault is this a good example of? *elongation due to angulation too low.*
        (b) What two techniques are available for obtaining intra-oral radiographs?
        (c) Compare the merits of each technique.

Bisecting   q   Paralleling.
① Size of image is   ① Size is nearer
   distorted.   to real + sharper.

② Can be done at   ② Only 70 kvp / 4
   50 kvp   more.

③ Short cone   ③ Long cone only.

④ No film holder   ④ Needs a film
                                holder.

⑤ more radiation   ⑤ Less radiation

⑥ Round collimation   ⑥ Rectangular
                                collimation.

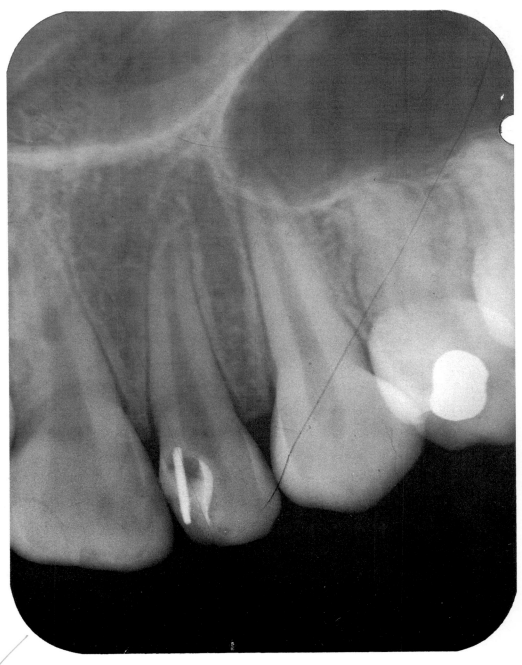

Q4.7   This patient was thought to have a periapical infection of ⌐2 .
(a) What radiographic features confirm the diagnosis?
(b) What radiographic feature is clearly shown? *y line of Ennis*
(mein section of lateral
nasal wall & floor of antrum)

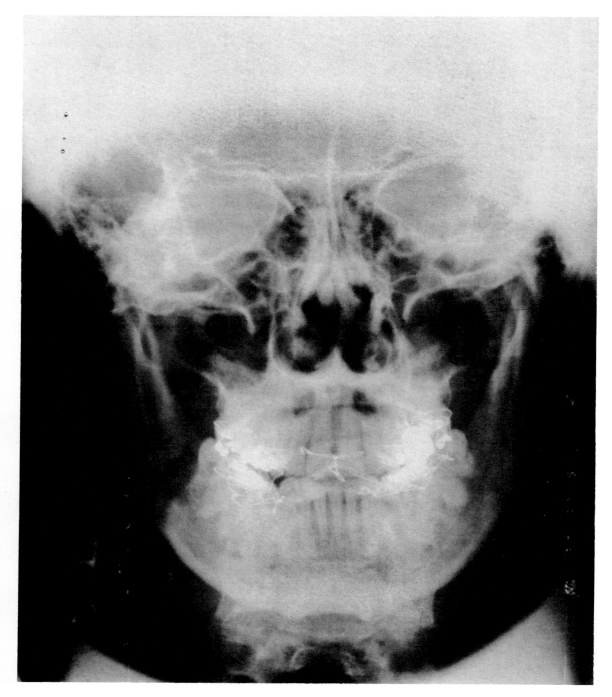

Q4.8   (a) This is a postero-anterior (PA) view of a patient with a fractured right angle of mandible that has been treated. How have the jaws been immobilized?

(b) Is there sufficient radiographic evidence in this view to indicate that all is well?

(c) What would be the indications for inserting an intra-osseous wire or plate to stabilize the fracture affecting the right mandibular angle?

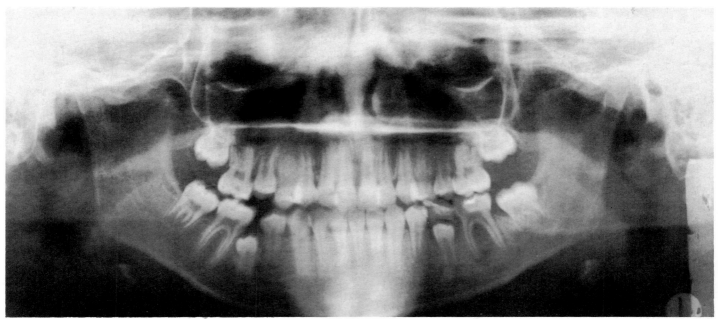

Extraction
of E
E

20% chance
that 8's will
develop

Q4.9   (a) What has been the likely past dental history of this patient?
         (b) What is the probability that the third molars will develop at this age?

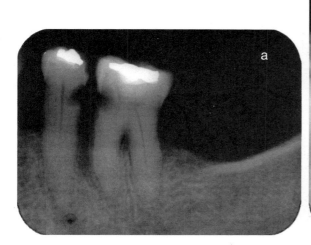

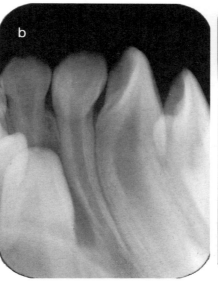

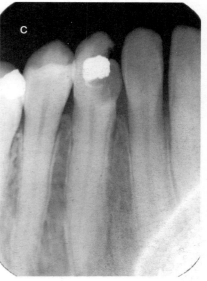

Film
upside down in
mouth

Q4.10   What is wrong with the technique used to take these various radiographs?

AOS pg. 80

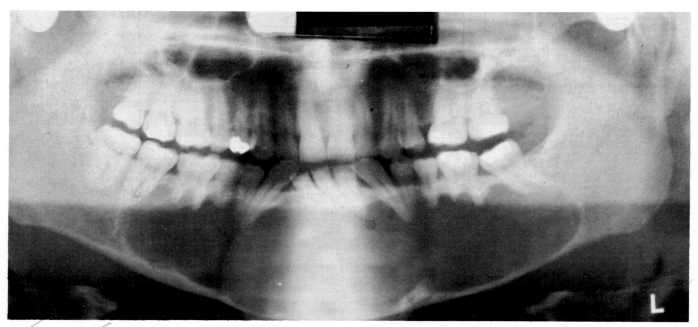

Q4.11 (a) What is the probable diagnosis?
(b) What treatment might be appropriate?

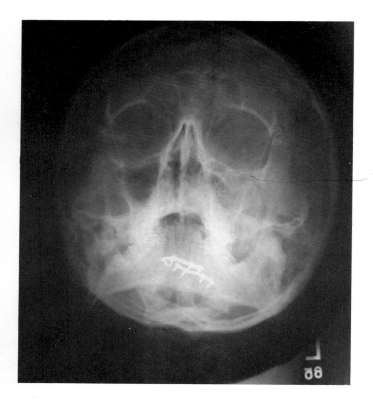

Q4.12 (a) What maxillo-facial fixation methods are shown in this radiograph? When are they indicated?
(b) The patient suffered a Le Fort II pattern of maxillary fracture and has fractured the left neck of condyle. In what order would you reduce the fractures and why?
(c) How important are radiographs in the investigation and diagnosis of the injuries illustrated here?

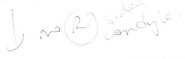

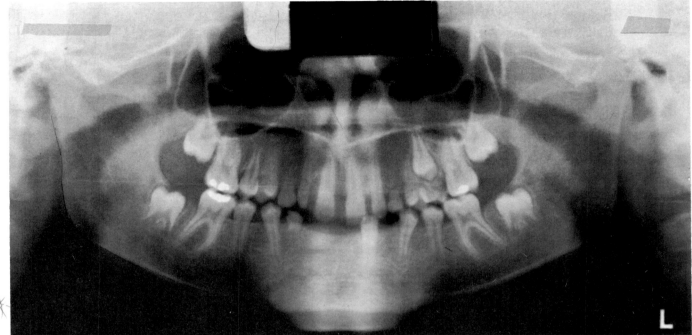

Q4.13 This is a 13 year old healthy female.
  (a) What abnormalities are present on the radiograph? Suggest a diagnosis.
  (b) Teeth may occasionally be absent in pantomographic views—why?

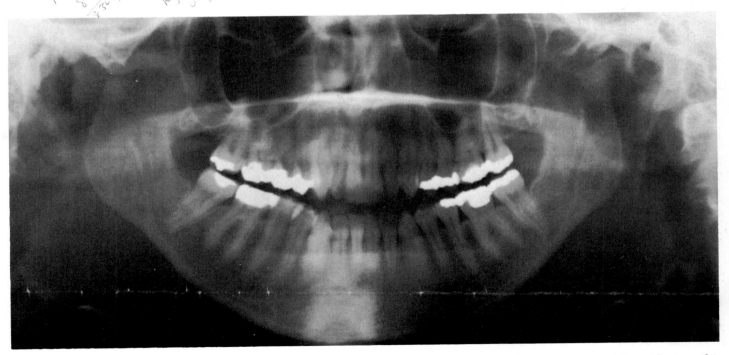

Q4.14 (a) Describe the main abnormalities apart from the anterior open bite evident on this pantomograph.
  (b) Is the pantomograph ideal for the radiographic assessment of temporomandibular joints?
  (c) What are the causes of anterior open bite?
  (d) In the absence of any progressive pathology, how would you manage this patient?

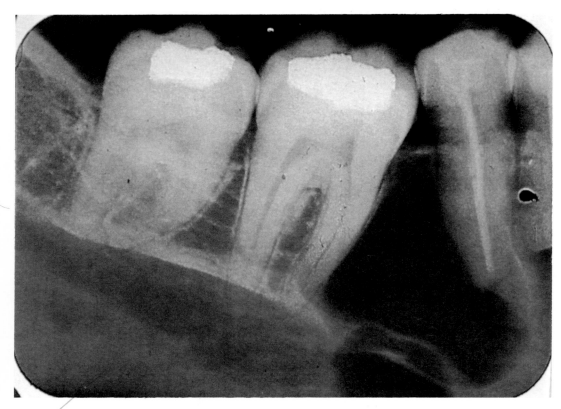

Q4.15   (a) What is the main problem?
          (b) From which tissue is this type of lesion thought to be derived?
          (c) What is the appropriate treatment?

pg. 86

PAPER 4 · ANSWERS

A4.1   (a) Mesioangular impaction of ⌐8. Over-extended MOD restoration of ⌐6, and recurrent caries in ⌐6.

     (b) (i) Angulation of the impacted tooth—estimated by examining the inclination of the occlusal surface of the impacted tooth with a line drawn along the occlusal surfaces of the first and second permanent molars.

         (ii) Bony covering of the tooth—this is the area beneath a line drawn from the surface of the alveolar bone distal to the impacted tooth to the bony septum between the first and second molars.

         (iii) Depth of application of the elevator—the distance from the bony surface to the point of application (usually the enamel–cementum junction on the mesial aspect of the impacted mesioangular tooth).

         (iv) Crown size, root morphology, and caries status of second and third molars.

         (v) Texture of investing bone of the impacted tooth.

         (vi) Location of the inferior alveolar nerve.

A4.2   (a) The child has amelogenesis imperfecta.

       The enamel of the crowns of all teeth is thin, has broken off, and has almost the same radiodensity as dentine. The patient does not have dentinogenesis imperfecta as all teeth have relatively normal roots and pulps. ✻ ✻

     (b) Autosomal dominant (see figure).

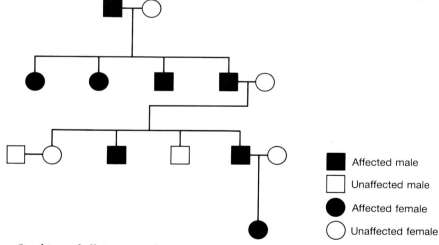

A4.3   (i) Stacking of all upper molars.

     (ii) Retained ECBA|BCDE
               EDCB|BCDE.

     (iii) Unerupted 85321| 23458
                 85432|234578.

     (iv) Partially erupted ⌐7; 7|7 may also be partially erupted.

     (v) Cysts (dentigerous) about 87|78.

     (vi) Caries E|DE
              |6.

     (vii) Unerupted supernumerary in ⌐12 area.

A4.4   (a) Parallax technique—two radiographs of the same structure are taken, each only differing in the horizontal angulation of the X-ray source.

(b) The canine is palatal to the dental arch.

If the canine appears to move in the same direction as the X-ray tube, the tooth lies palatal to the arch; if it moves in the opposite direction the tooth lies buccal to the arch.

To demonstrate the parallax effect place one hand in front of the other at the level of your nose. Move your head to the right—the hand nearest your nose will seem to move to the left while the other hand will seem to move to the right.

A4.5   (a) There is a generalized loss of periodontal bone.

(b) Several systemic disorders have now been associated with increased susceptibility to periodontal breakdown. The increased periodontitis arises either because of reduced oral hygiene measures, reduced host immunity, or alterations in bio-chemical or anatomical features of the periodontium. For example:

Impaired oral hygiene
Handicapping disorders (both physical and mental)
Facial palsies
Xerostomia.

Immunodeficiency
Leukaemia
Neutropenia
Agranulocytosis
Insulin-dependent diabetes mellitus
HIV infection
Chediak–Higashi syndrome (rare)
Acatalasia (rare)
Papillon–Lefevre syndrome (rare)
Crohn's disease (not proven).

Anatomical abnormalities (Biochemical/anatomical defects)
Ehlers–Danlos syndrome, sub-type VIII (rare)
Hypophosphataemia (rare)
Dentine dysplasia, Shield's type I (rare).

A4.6   (a) This film was taken using the bisecting angle technique—the angulation of the X-ray cone was too low, hence there is elongation of the images. There is also a mark left by the incorrect mounting of the film during drying.

(b) (i) Bisecting angle technique—the X-ray beam is directed perpendicular to an imaginary plane that bisects the angle between the long axis of the tooth and the plane of the dental film. Ideally this ensures that the radiographic image has the exact dimensions of the object. In the bisecting angle technique the film is not parallel to the object.

     (ii) Long-cone paralleling technique—the plane of the film is parallel to the long axis of the tooth and the X-ray beam is directed perpendicular to both object and film.

(c) The bisecting angle technique can be undertaken using a 'conventional' low-kilovoltage (eg 50 kV) dental X-ray unit, but the long source-to-film distance of the long-cone paralleling technique necessitates the use of a higher kilovoltage (eg 70 kV) X-ray unit. In addition, special film holders are required for the latter technique.

Long cone paralleling allows rectangular collimation, hence residual radiation is minimized.

Sharper and more accurate images of teeth and periodontal bone can probably be obtained by the long-cone paralleling technique, but as this procedure requires accurate parallel alignment of the film with the tooth it may take longer than the bisecting angle technique.

A4.7 (a) There is a discontinuity of the lamina dura on the mesial aspect of the apex of $\underline{2}$.

(b) The Y formation (or sign) of Ennis—this is the area of intersection of the lateral margin of the nasal floor and the floor of the maxillary antrum.

A4.8 (a) Eyelet wiring and intermaxillary fixation.

Eyelet wires are made from 0.4 to 0.6 mm gauge stainless steel wire pre-stretched by 10 per cent. Eyelet wiring is effective for immobilizing jaw fractures of dentate patients, where tooth spacing is not a feature (as in this case). Where many teeth are absent, other methods of fixation, such as arch bars, are more applicable.

Eyelet wires can be easily applied to most teeth, although the conical shape and position of some third molars and lower canines can present problems. The wires may be applied to lone-standing molars by passing both loops around the tooth. A single eyelet wire may also be passed around more than two teeth and this technique is useful close to fracture lines, for example in the lower incisor region.

(b) A lateral radiographic view is also required to check for adequate reduction in the sagittal plane. The pantomograph (Fig. A4.8) illustrates that while the reduction is adequate it is not ideal as there is a step deformity at the lower border. A lateral oblique view would also illustrate displacement in this plane. In cases such as this, muscle pull will tend to displace the posterior segment medially, and this displacement may not be apparent on a pantomograph, particularly if the fracture is horizontally favourable. Both PA and lateral views are therefore needed, but it must be remembered that radiographic assessment of fractures should always follow thorough clinical examination.

(c) Indications for intra-osseous wiring or bone plates (e.g., Champy plates) include instability of the posterior segment, particularly where the mandible is fractured posterior to the last standing molar. Upper border wires are easily inserted if a

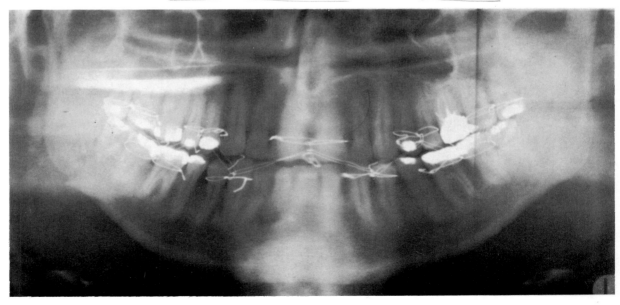

Fig. A4.8

third molar is removed at the time of operation, but lower border wires generally give a more stable and secure result, especially where comminution is a feature at the upper border. However, the latter technique has disadvantages—such as the necessity for a general anaesthetic and for an external approach, damage to the facial nerve and artery, and stripping of periosteum—which can give rise to delayed union in elderly patients.

A4.9   (a) Early loss of E|
                     E|.

E| was removed rather earlier than E|. This has allowed the 6| to move mesially. This in turn has provided additional space for the 7|, which has therefore erupted rather earlier than the contralateral tooth. E| was probably lost only a few months before this radiograph was obtained as there is relatively little space loss for the 5|.

(b) As the patient is aged 12 to 13 years and there is no sign of the third molars, there is only about a 20 per cent chance that these molars will now develop.

A4.10   (a) The film has been placed upside down in the mouth such that the locating mark was directly adjacent to the apex of |5, thus radiographic confirmation of periapical periodontitis may be hampered.

(b) The film has been bent while the radiograph was taken.

(c) The film and/or X-ray source has been malpositioned such that the apices of the teeth have been missed and the images elongated.

A4.11   (a) 2| is absent from the lower dental arch such that 1|123 have tilted to the right. There is a large radiolucency of the body of mandible extending from 7| to |7. There is a lower incisor lying on the intact inferior border of the mandible below |3. The radiolucency is possibly a very large dentigerous cyst.

(b) Histopathological examination of the cyst lining is essential to confirm the diagnosis. Large cysts can be treated either by enucleation or marsupilization. In view of the large size of this lesion, marsupialization via an incision in the lower labial sulcus might be most appropriate. The cavity should be initially packed with ribbon gauze containing an antiseptic—such as Whitehead's varnish. After a few weeks this pack should be removed and either replaced with a smaller one or with an acrylic bung fitted to ensure patency of the hole in the labial vestibule. The lining can be completely removed once the cyst has shrunk to a suitably small size. It is important to note that the vitality of all the lower teeth should be determined and any non-vital teeth treated by orthograde root-canal filling before surgery or retrograde filling at time of surgery.

A4.12   (a) (i) *Fronto-zygomatic 'figure of eight' wire.* This method of fixation is indicated where there has been separation or fracture of the fronto-zygomatic suture, and when there is instability following reduction. Simplicity of insertion and the cosmetic advantage of invasion in the supra-orbital region makes this a particularly suitable method of stabilizing a fracture of the zygomatic complex. The 'figure of eight' wire produces stability in all three planes, whereas a simple loop tends to give stability in only two planes.

(ii) *Infra-orbital (zygomatic–maxillary) wire.* Wiring in this region may be necessary to immobilize a fracture of the zygomatic complex. However, fronto-zygomatic wiring on its own is often sufficient in most cases of instability unless there are functional or cosmetic problems. Discontinuity of the infra-orbital rim *per se* is not an indication for open (or even closed) reduction. Exploration of the orbital floor, for example when there is interference with the inferior rectus or inferior oblique muscle function, or enophthalmos, may provide an opportunity to restore a comminuted orbital rim to anatomical form by means of an intra-osseous wire.

(iii) *Interdental eyelet wires.* Though the use of direct rigid fixation (e.g., plates) obviates the need for intermaxillary fixation (IMF), eyelet wiring continues to be widely used in many cases of mandibular and maxillary fractures. IMF is a simple, inexpensive, and effective method in dentate patients with a good complement of teeth. Eyelet wires may be used to obtain stability across a fracture site, may be adapted for use on lone-standing molar teeth, and can be inserted under local anaesthesia or sedation without local anaesthesia. Archbars are more suitable where the teeth are spaced, when several teeth are missing, or when elastic traction is required.

(iv) *'Champy' plates.* Two Champy plates have been used to stabilize a symphyseal fracture. They are recognizable as such because they have been adapted to bony contours, are narrow between screw-holes, and have relatively short

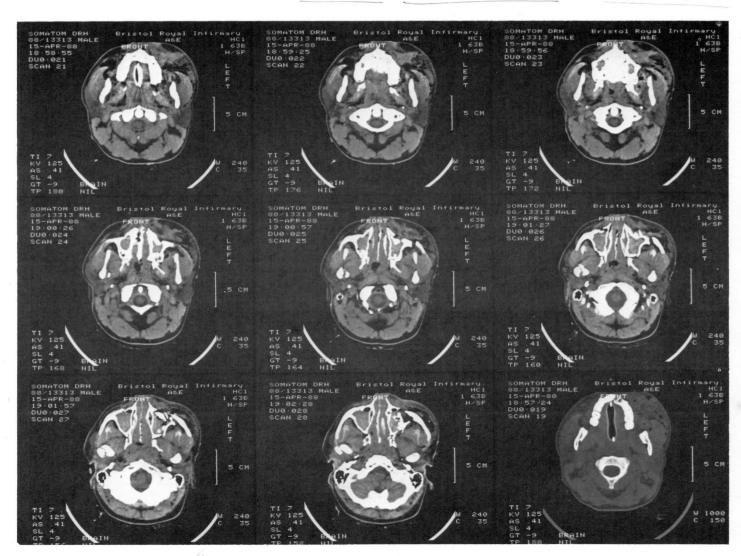

Fig. A4.12 Axial computed tomographic views of the same patient showing fractures of the left maxillary, naso-ethmoidal, and zygomatic regions.

screws engaging only the buccal cortex. Plating of maxillo-facial fractures can be carried out at virtually any accessible bony site, though the neck of the mandible is difficult. Plating is particularly useful in fixation of mid-face osteotomies, and has largely superseded the more modified internal suspension and external pin-fixation techniques.

(b) Two important principles of management should be applied. The mandible should normally be reconstructed first. This provides a reference (the lower teeth) for the reduction of the Le Fort II fracture. If the mid-face fractures were reduced first, the occlusion would almost certainly be incorrect as maxillary bone is often crushed or comminuted. Furthermore, when one condyle is fractured, allowance must be made for shortening of the ramus on the ipsilateral side, and it is therefore important to initially consider restoring the occlusal plane.

After mandibular reconstruction, disimpaction, and reduction of the maxillary fracture should be preceded by reduction of the fractured zygomatic complex, otherwise it may not be possible to fully reduce the Le Fort II segment and asymmetry will result. It is also important to check facial symmetry, particularly the zygomatic prominences, as reduction of the Le Fort II fracture may be accompanied by movement in the reduced zygoma.

Though the application of these principles usually leads to a satisfactory result, precise restoration of the facial skeleton to its original form requires an appreciation of possible discrepancies in all three planes. If closed reduction seems unsatisfactory, open reduction should be considered. Relatives are often able to provide photographs, which give useful information for correct facial reconstruction.

(c) The relative importance of clinical examination and radiographic findings in the diagnosis of fractures varies according to site, ease of examination, and patient co-operation. Superimposition of images and the two-dimensional nature of all radiographs are important limitations. Over-reliance on radiographs leads to mistakes in diagnosis, particularly with regard to symphyseal fractures in the mandible and to high-level maxillary fractures where adequate clinical examination is of paramount important (e.g., the Le Fort II fracture is not particularly evident here). Gentle but determined efforts should be made to detect mobility in these areas, particularly by applying pressure to the teeth across suspected fracture sites. The orbital margins should be thoroughly palpated. Intra-oral haematomas can also be important signs of underlying bony injury. Supplementary information is then used to confirm or refute clinical impressions and to provide details of injury, for example, to the orbital, pterygoid plate and naso-ethmoid regions (Fig. A4.12).

A4.13 (a) (i) Absence of $\underline{83\quad|\quad 38}$
$8321|138$.

(ii) Unerupted $\underline{|5}$ and $\underline{7|7}$
$7|7$.

(iii) Retained $\underline{C|C}$
$C|\quad$.

The diagnosis would be hypodontia (oligodontia) with retention of $|E$ and delayed eruption of $|5$.

(b) Pantomographic systems are so designed always to obtain an image of a slice of the body at the same depth in all patients. However, the slice may miss a tooth-bearing area, and hence teeth can appear to be absent. Never rely on radiographs alone, *always examine the patient*.

A4.14 (a) This pantomograph demonstrates absence of the right mandibular condyle and severe resorption of the left condyle. Loss of cortical outline is also a feature and, though the mouth does not appear to be open, the right mandibular condyle remnant lies anterior to the glenoid fossa. On the left side, there is 'lipping' of the condyle anteriorly and an irregular appearance of the rest of the articular surface. The radio-opacity affecting the mid part of the articular surface may represent an osteophyte or even ankylosis. An anterior open bite is also evident.

This patient in fact had suffered from osteoarthritis of the temporomandibular joint for many years and bilateral condylectomies had been performed. The condyles were serially removed over a two-year period, five years before this OPT. Though she derived some benefit from these operations (the anterior open bite did

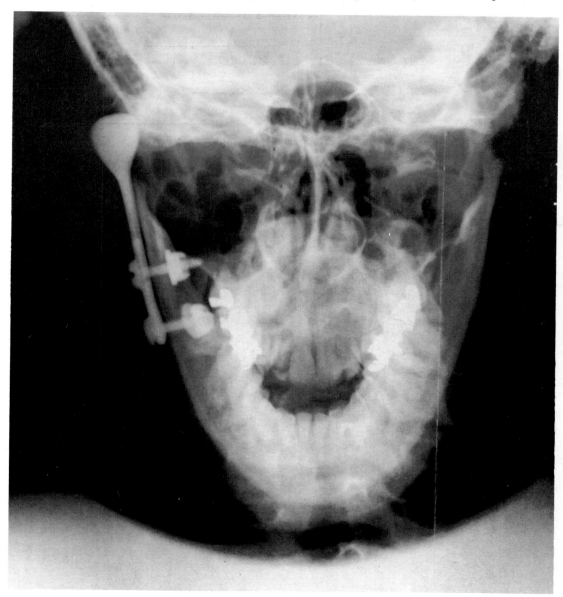

Fig. A4.14

not develop after surgery), a subsequent course of high-dose prednisolone for colitis gave rise to crippling occlusal problems secondary to further resorption and shortening of the ramus bilaterally and the development of an anterior open bite. It then became necessary to reconstruct both temporomandibular joints.

(b) Although the pantomograph is a good screening film for pathology of the temporomandibular joint, it suffers from all the disadvantages of tomographic techniques, including loss of definition and uneven image magnification. In addition some aspects of the joint may not fall within the 'trough' brought into focus by any particular machine. Plain films, such as transpharyngeal or transcranial views, are therefore often required to give further information.

(c) Anterior open bite may represent a congenital deformity, sometimes secondary to increased facial height or a skeletal Class III basal-bone relationship. Disorders of growth such as condylar hypertrophy may give rise to anterior open bite; in the case of a unilateral hyperplasia, this will be lateral as well as anterior. In an established case, where the hyperplastic process has ceased, occlusal compensation may eliminate the anterior open bite.

Acromegaly may also give rise to anterior open bite and the patient may demonstrate typical abnormalities of the extremities and cranium. Diagnosis in these growth-related problems is made largely through the history and clinical examination. Scintiscanning and growth hormone levels may confirm the clinical findings.

Other causes of anterior open bite include bilateral condylar dislocation, and bilateral fractures affecting the mandibular condyles, angles, or body of the mandible. Habits such as thumb-sucking may also give rise to this problem.

(d) In this patient, resorption of the condyles ceased after resolution of the colitis and cessation of corticosteroid therapy. Reconstruction was undertaken to restore the posterior height of the mandible in a way least likely to give rise to further bony resorption. Though bilateral costo-chondral grafts could have been used, it was thought that more durable fixation would be an advantage and alloplastic materials (Fig. A4.14) were therefore used. On the right side a Bowerman–Conroy titanium condylar prosthesis was screwed to the ascending ramus. On the left side, in view of the additional bone available, an ulnar head prosthesis was inserted. This silastic prosthesis appears to be particularly suitable for cases of ankylosis, having a central core that can easily insert into the medulla of the residual condyle neck, and an articular surface with a large surface area.

A4.15 (a) Cystic radiolucency in the $\overline{75}$ region, probably a radicular cyst associated with the root of $\overline{5}$ or a residual cyst related to $\overline{6}$ (now extracted).

(b) Radicular cysts are thought to be derived from epithelial rests of Malassez. The exact stimulus for proliferation is not known; however, possible stimuli may be derived from invading micro-organisms or from the associated immune response.

(c) Check the vitality of $\overline{7}$: if $\overline{7}$ is non-vital, this will require orthograde root-canal therapy. In addition, apicectomy and a retrograde root filling of $\overline{5}$ with enucleation of the associated cyst will be necessary. This surgery may be complicated by the presence of the mental nerve. To avoid unnecessary damage, the mental nerve must be identified and protected before bone removal.

PAPER 5 · QUESTIONS

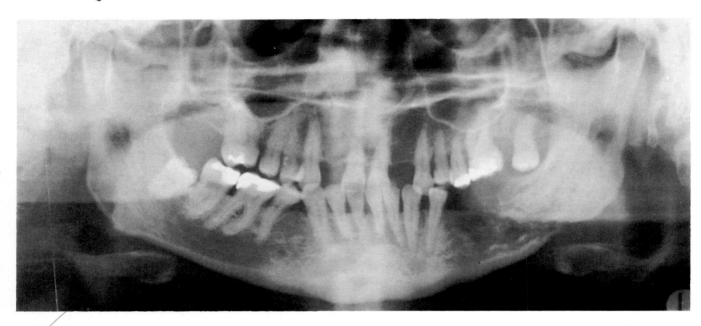

Q5.1 This patient had radiotherapy for a carcinoma of the left side of the tongue and floor of mouth.
(a) What has happened to the left body of the mandible?
(b) What is the differential diagnosis?
(c) How can this be treated?

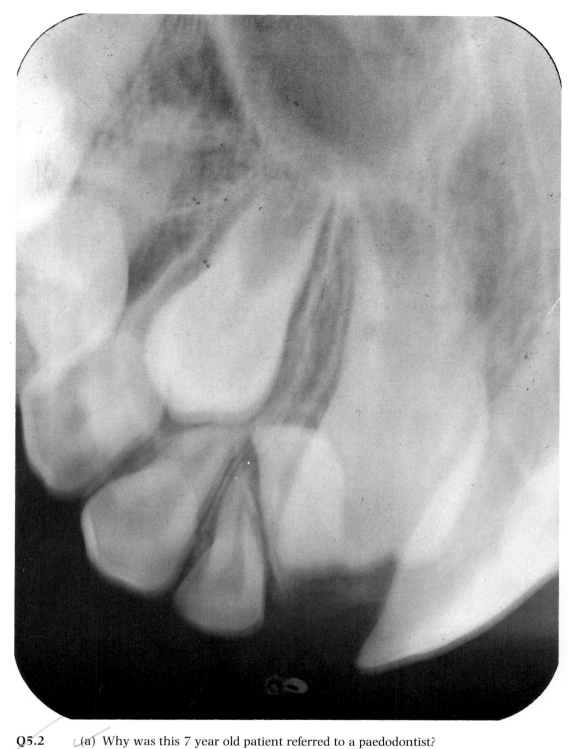

Q5.2 (a) Why was this 7 year old patient referred to a paedodontist?
(b) How can the lesion be localized?

Pg - 107   Ocel view

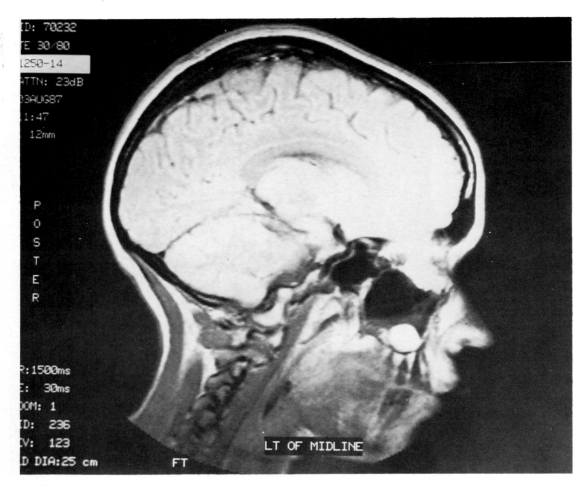

Q5.3 (a) What technique has been employed to obtain this image?
        (b) What differentiates images obtained in this way from radiographic computerized tomographic images?
        (c) What applications may this technique have in the investigation of orofacial disease?

(Courtesy of Heinemann Medical Books)

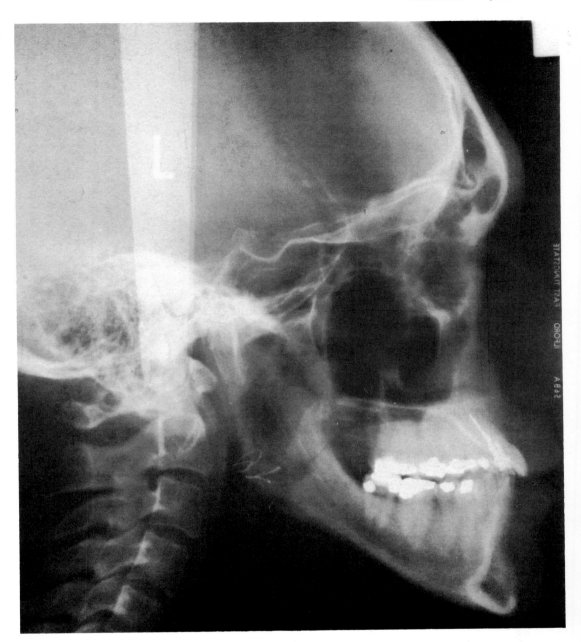

Q5.4   Give an appraisal of the post-operative radiograph of this patient who has had orthognathic surgery.

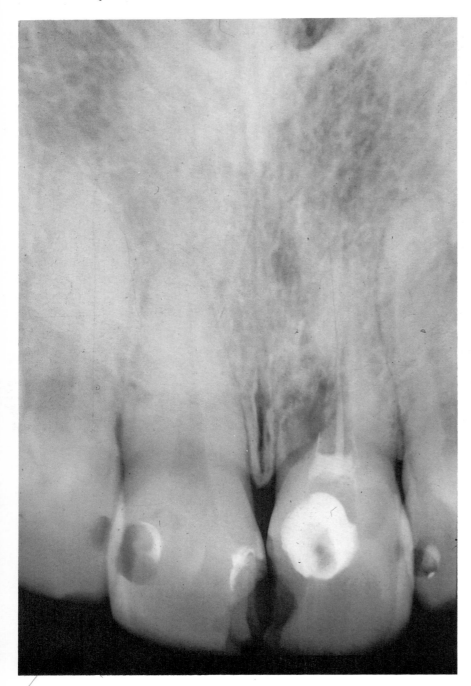

Q5.5   This 18 year old male patient complains of increasing looseness of an upper front tooth.
(a) Provide a diagnosis.
(b) What is the likely cause of the problem?
(c) List other causes of this disorder.
(d) How might you manage this patient?

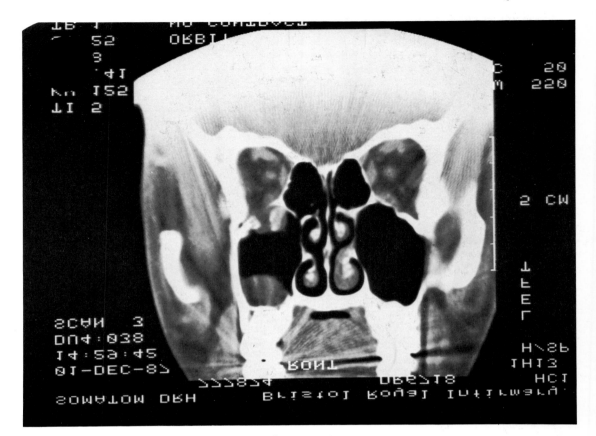

Q5.6   This 25 year old man received a blow to the right side of the face.
  (a) Which injuries are shown on this coronal computerized tomograph?
  (b) What is the likely effect if the injury is not treated?
  (c) What radiographic views are usually required for the routine radiographic assessment of a possible fracture of the zygomatic complex?

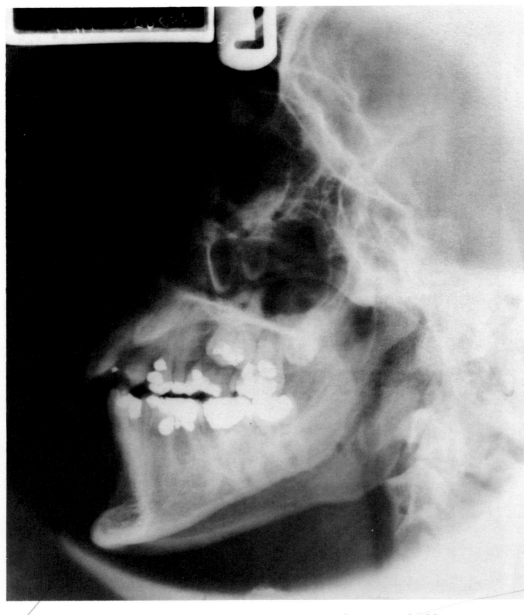

Q5.7   This 35 year old female with systemic lupus erythematosus had been receiving prednisolone (10 mg daily) for the past two years.
(a) What abnormality is present?
(b) What special precautions are required in relation to oral surgery?

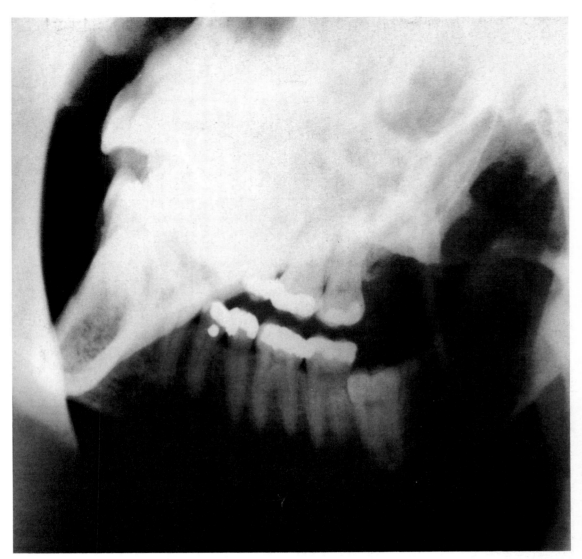

Q5.8   This left oblique lateral X-ray shows a slightly mesio-angular impacted ⌐8, in a 35 year old female.
(a) What hazards are involved in the removal of this tooth?
(b) What precautions should be taken to avoid these?

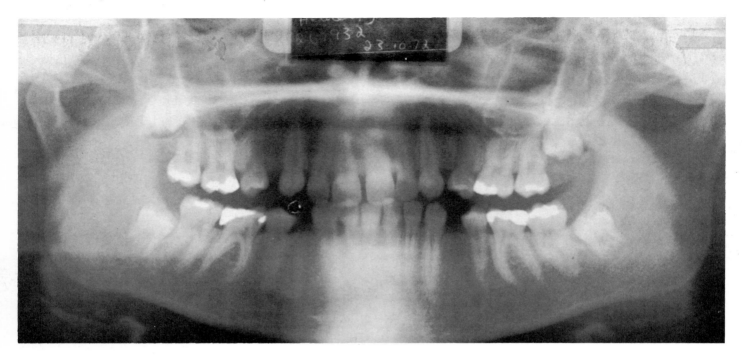

Q5.9   (a) Is the centre-line discrepancy shown here between the upper and lower arches of any orthodontic significance?

(b) Has the loss of all four first premolars in any way altered the chance of third molars erupting?

(c) What is the radio-opacity in the upper left premolar region?

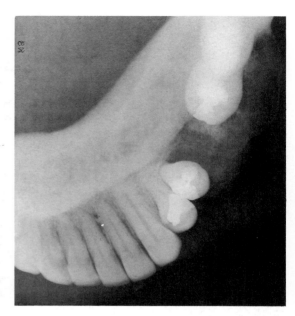

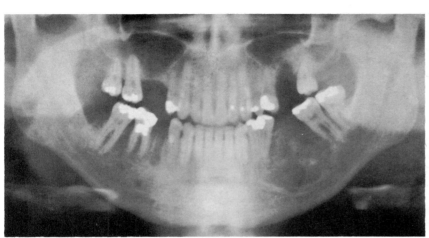

Q5.10   (a) Describe the radiographic abnormalities shown in these two films from the same patient.
         (b) What is the differential diagnosis?

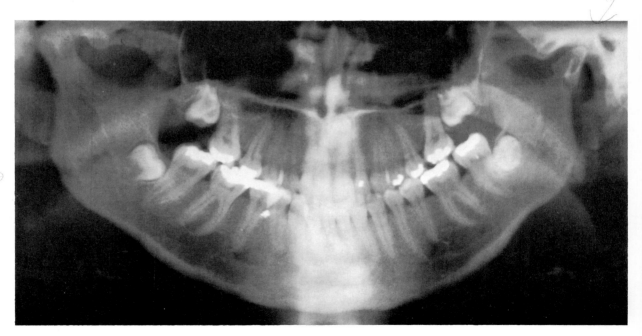

Q5.11   (a) The patient was punched in the face—are there any fractures visible on this radiograph?
         (b) What, if any, management is required?

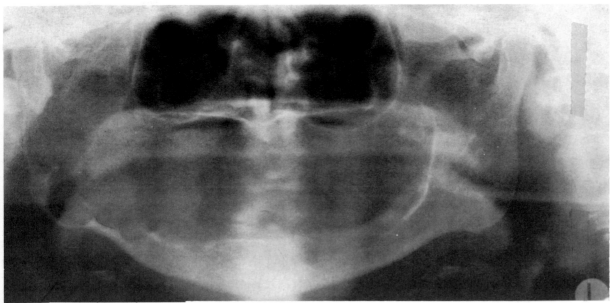

Q5.12   (a) What abnormality is present? Suggest a diagnosis.
         (b) What additional investigations may help confirm the diagnosis?

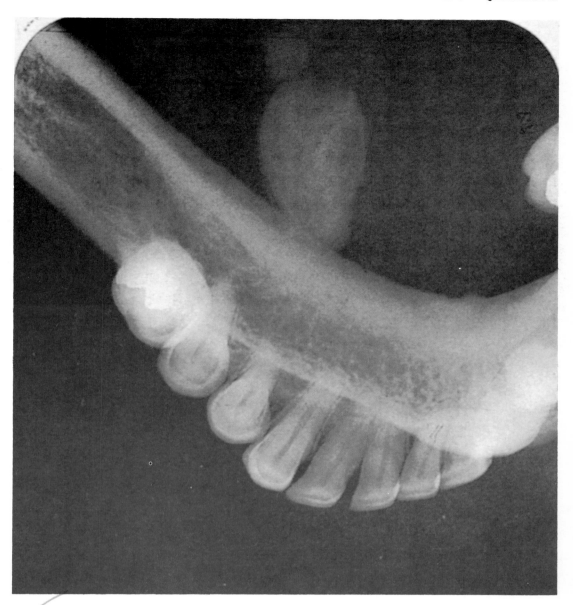

Q5.13   This patient complained of a burning pain in his mouth each time he ate.
(a) What is the diagnosis?
(b) What are the main clinical features of this disorder?
(c) What is the treatment of this condition?

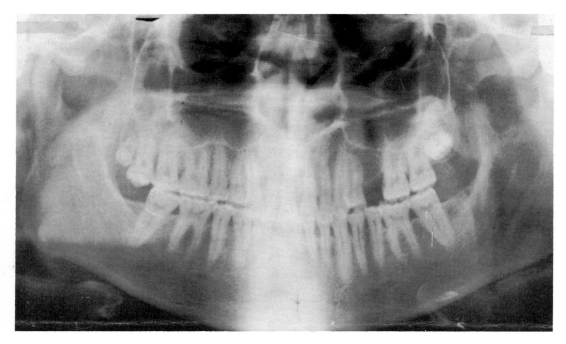

Q5.14   This patient has had both lower third molars extracted.
(a) What dental anomalies are present?
(b) What treatment may be required?
(c) Where do supplemental teeth usually occur?

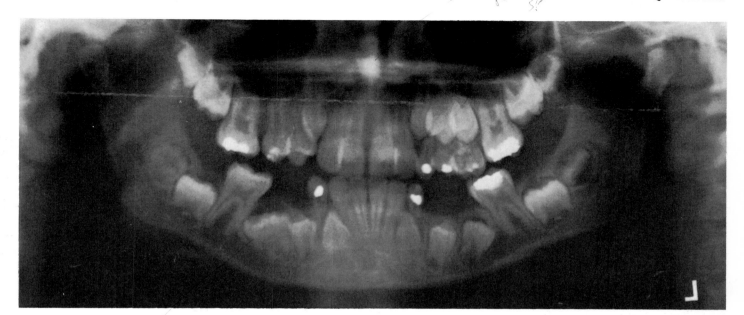

Q5.15 (a) Is the form of the ⎺5⏋ truly macrodont or is this appearance due to the patient moving during the exposure?

(b) What is the radio-opacity at the level of the floor of the nose above the apices of the maxillary central incisors?

PAPER 5 · ANSWERS

A5.1   (a) Osteoradionecrosis has progressed to the extent where a spontaneous (pathological) fracture has occurred.

(b) The radiolucencies in the mandible could be due to tumour deposits.
    The radiographic appearances of osteoradionecrosis frequently cannot be distinguished from osteomyelitis, but the latter is usually associated with frank suppuration. The necrotic bone of osteoradionecrosis resembles soggy, rotten wood, is often visible in the mouth, and appears dark brown or black.

(c) Small areas of osteoradionecrosis can spontaneously sequester but, if there are large areas involved, as here, or there is recurrent secondary osteomyelitis or likely pathological fracture, the only possible treatment is to resect the mandible, extending anteriorly and posteriorly until bleeding bone is reached. Provided the site heals with intact mucosal cover, the mandible can be grafted with vital bone. Inert materials may lead to a recurrence of infection. In this patient a partial mandibulectomy achieved mucosal cover but a small sinus remained, draining pus externally below the operative site. The patient died from a massive haemorrhage due to erosion of a pharyngeal artery by tumour.

A5.2   (a) There is delayed eruption of 1| due to the presence of a radio-opacity associated with the crown of 1|. The radio-opacity is most likely to be a supernumerary tooth. 2| is absent.

(b) (i) Palpation of the labial and palatal aspects of 1|.

(ii) Parallax views of the 1| region—occlusal views are less likely to be useful (Fig. A5.2).

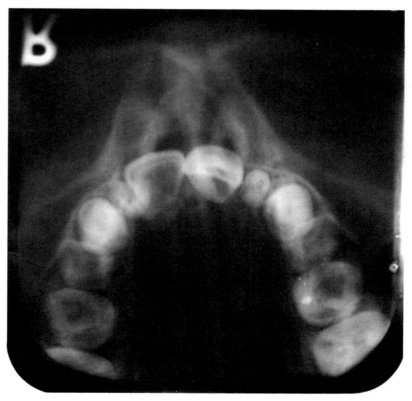

Fig. A5.2   The occlusal view of 1| failed to reveal the precise location of the supernumerary tooth.

A5.3   (a) Magnetic resonance imaging (MRI). In this technique a strong magnetic field causes the alignment of nuclei, and then radio-frequency electromagnetic waves are used to deflect this alignment. When the radio-frequency waves are stopped, the atoms realign themselves, releasing electromagnetic energy—which is the energy that is detected.

              Hydrogen nuclei are most easily imaged, and as most hydrogen is present as water, MRI principally detects tissues containing large amounts of water (soft tissues mainly).

      (b) As MRI principally detects water-containing tissues, the teeth and bone will *not* be clearly demonstrated. In computerized tomography (CT) calcified structures *can* be imaged.

      (c) There have been few reports of the application of MRI to orofacial disease. However, it may have application in the investigation of:

          Mucosal abnormalities of the sinuses and pharynx

          Muscles of the infratemporal fossa and soft palate

          Salivary gland neoplasms (MRI does not visualize calcifications—but it may be possible to identify branches of the facial nerve)

          Oral carcinoma and other neoplasms—as metal dental restorations and appliances do not disrupt image quality, MRI may be more applicable than CT in the investigation of orofacial neoplasms and in radiation field planning

          Localization of enlarged lymph nodes in the neck and determination of their relationship to large blood vessels and nerves

          Disease of the temporomandibular joint.

A5.4   This is the same patient as in Q3.13.

              A very acceptable profile and occlusion has been achieved by a vertical sub-sigmoid osteotomy alone. The set-back has been supplemented by a slight increase in the lower face height (55 per cent), which has produced an average maxillary/mandibular plane angle. Note that, despite this increase in lower face height, the lip coverage is still adequate.

              There remains a moderate residual skeletal class III dental-base relationship (ANB = 4.5°) but this is offset by the original lower incisor retroclination and upper incisor proclination, which has been retained. This has allowed a Class I incisor occlusion to be achieved on what is still a skeletal III base.

A5.5   (a) External root resorption.

      (b) The patient most likely received a blow to his upper teeth in childhood. This may have caused concussion, subluxation, or luxation of the tooth.

      (c) Other causes of external root resorption include:

          Chronic mechanical trauma; for example—

              excessive orthodontic forces

              excessive traumatic occlusion

              cysts (e.g. radicular)

              trauma

              impacted teeth (e.g. lower third molars)

          Chemical trauma, e.g., root-canal medicaments (rare)

          Periapical infection

          Idiopathic

          Systemic (rare).

      (d) In view of the severity of the resorption, removal of the tooth seems necessary. Had there only been slight resorption, root-canal therapy with calcium hydroxide or an antibiotic/corticosteroid paste before root filling with gutta percha might have been considered appropriate by some clinicians.

A5.6   (a) This film has been specially produced to show soft tissues more clearly. A segment of the right orbital floor has dropped into the antrum and the inferior rectus/oblique muscle appears to be caught in the hole.

(b) This type of injury often results in inferior tethering of the eyeball and diplopia (double vision).

    The injury was treated by exploration of the orbital floor, elevation of the soft tissues from the defect, and insertion of a thin sheet of silastic to cover the hole. This corrected the visual problem.

(c) (i) 30° occipito-mental view—this shows the anterior margins of the orbital floors and the roof of the maxillary antra.

    (ii) 45° (basic) occipito-mental view—this demonstrates the bony margins of the maxillary antra and the zygomatic arches.

    (iii) Submento-vertex (SMV) view—this demonstrates the base of skull and the zygomatic buttresses and arches; it can also show the anterior mandible (Fig. A5.6). The SMV view is particularly useful for demonstrating the degree of zygomatic arch depression, but it must not be taken if there is any likelihood of damage to the cervical spine.

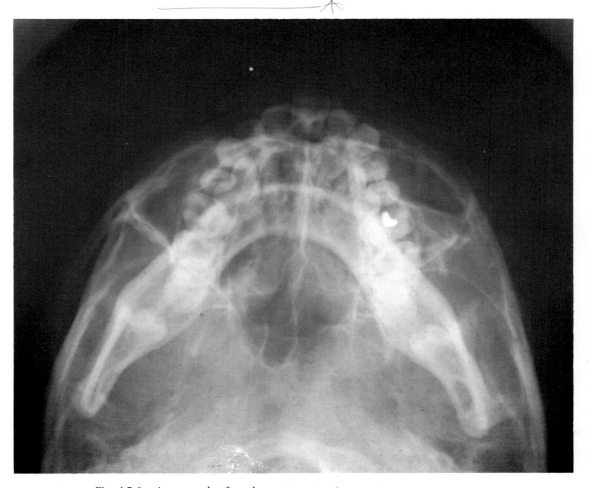

Fig. A5.6   An example of a submento-vertex view.

A5.7   (a) (i) Submerged $\lfloor 6$.

            (ii) Unerupted $\lfloor 8$.

(b) This patient has been receiving long-term corticosteroid therapy, thus steroid cover is required to minimize a possibly hypotensive event. One regimen is 200 mg hydrocortisone given intravenously immediately pre-operatively. The blood pressure should be monitored.

A5.8   (a) The tooth has a very small follicle space, no doubt related to the age of the patient, and there is a dark line across the root at the level of the mandibular canal suggesting that the root is grooved by the inferior alveolar nerve. There is very little mandible below the root of the tooth. Thus, anaesthesia of the inferior alveolar nerve and fracture of the mandible are possible hazards of the surgical removal of this tooth.

(b) As the lower third molar is more commonly grooved by the nerve on the lingual side, bone removal should be carried out accordingly to allow the tooth to move away from the nerve during its removal. It is important to remove sufficient bone to allow elevation with minimal force lest the mandible be fractured.

A5.9   (a) Patients often move their mandible slightly to one side when occluding edge-to-edge during the taking of a pantomograph. In this radiograph the difference between the position of the condyle on the articular eminence of each side and differences in the distances between the posterior border of each ramus and the body of C1 strongly suggest a lateral displacement of the mandible. On clinical examination with the patient in centric occlusion, the centre lines were coincident.

(b) Studies have shown that loss of any posterior tooth, including first premolars, reduces the incidence of lower third molar impaction.

(c) A retained root: almost certainly the mesial root of $\lfloor E$.

A5.10   (a) Both films demonstrate a well-defined radiolucency with patchy radio-opacity in the left body of the mandible. $\lceil 6$ is missing and there is no evidence of the socket. The lamina dura is absent from the distal surface of $\lceil 5$ and the mesial aspect of $\lceil 7$; the roots of both these teeth have been displaced. The inferior alveolar neurovascular bundle may have been displaced inferiorly, but the lesion does not appear to extend beyond it. The occlusal view shows both buccal and lingual expansion of the mandible, and diffuse multifocal radio-opacities within the body of the lesion.

(b) (i) Central ossifying fibroma of bone (central fibro-osteoma) is virtually always demarcated, in contrast to fibrous dysplasia. The lesion here is a long-standing one because calcification is very evident. In early ossifying fibromas, radio-lucency without radiopacity is more likely. Displacement of teeth is common in this lesion.

     (ii) Central cementifying fibroma shares all the above radiographic features, and radiologically is extremely difficult to differentiate from central ossifying fibroma. In addition, both these lesions can cause expansion of the mandible in all planes and radiographically the outline of the expanded cortex is continuous with the outline of the lesion within the mandible. The only real accepted difference is histological in that the ossifying fibroma involves osteoblast proliferation and new bone formation, and in the cementifying fibroma cementoblasts proliferate with cementum formation.

     (iii) Fibrous dysplasia gives rise to similar radiographic features. It may present as a well-defined mono- or multilocular radiolucency with or without patchy opacities. More established, longstanding cases exhibit a less well-defined radio-opacity that has a classic 'ground-glass' appearance not evident in either of the views illustrated. This ground-glass appearance is usually uniform. Teeth can be displaced but rarely is there root resorption.

(iv) Paget's disease (osteitis deformans) affects the maxilla more commonly than the mandible and the 'cotton-wool' appearance of the affected bone is less well defined. Again the radiographic appearance depends upon the stage of the disease: early Paget's disease may give rise to discrete radiolucencies that precede osteoblastic activity. Paget's disease usually affects the skeleton bilaterally.

(v) Sclerosing osteomyelitis gives rise to diffuse radio-opacity within the mandible and, like Paget's disease, (but unlike the other lesions listed) can give rise to labial paraesthesia.

A5.11   (a) Fracture of the neck of the left condyle.

(b) The occlusion is undisturbed and therefore reduction of the fracture and immobilization are not indicated.

     The patient should be advised to have a soft diet and avoid any excess mouth opening for 10 to 14 days. The patient should be reviewed clinically for the next 6 to 12 weeks to ensure the occlusion is maintained and that correct function has returned.

A5.12   (a) There is a large multilocular radiolucency of the right ramus and angle of the mandible. In view of its radiographic appearance and position the lesion is probably either an ameloblastoma or an odontogenic keratocyst.

(b) (i) Aspiration and examination of any cyst fluid. Fluid is unlikely to be obtained if the lesion is an ameloblastoma, whereas if it is a keratocyst, fluid with a protein concentration of less than 4 g/100 ml may be obtained. However, if the cyst has become infected, the protein concentration may be higher than 4 g/100 ml and, thus the profile of cyst fluid is not always an accurate diagnostic test.

(ii) Biopsy of lesional tissue. This can be carried out under local analgesia before any elective surgery.

(iii) Postero-anterior views of the lesion may allow detection of any buccal or lingual expansion.

(iv) Computed tomography might be of value to determine if there has been spread into adjacent soft tissues.

A5.13   (a) Submandibular calculus (sialolithiasis).

(b) At mealtimes the affected gland rapidly becomes swollen and patients suffer a burning-like pain localized to the floor of the mouth and submandibular area. The swelling and pain only diminish when all salivatory stimuli have been removed.

(c) A second radiograph, at 90° to the occlusal plane, should be taken to aid localization of the calculus. If the calculus lies (as in this patient) within the duct or anterior part of the gland, a simple incision in the floor of the mouth can be made and the calculus removed. The incision should be parallel to the submandibular duct. However, if the calculus lies in the infraposterior part of the submandibular gland, complete removal of the gland via an extra-oral approach may be required.

A5.14   (a) (i) Unerupted ⌊8.

(ii) Supplemental tooth distal to 8⌋.

(b) Due to the lack of opposing teeth, 98| may over-erupt and traumatize the adjacent buccal mucosa. In addition, over-eruption of 8| may cause food-trapping between 87|, thus predisposing to caries and/or periodontal disease. Thus removal of 98| is indicated. |8 is unerupted and not in communication with the mouth—thus unless it erupts further, removal of |8 is *not* indicated.

(c) In Europeans, supplemental teeth are rare and are seen mainly in the upper lateral incisor and lower incisor regions, while in black Africans and Orientals the premolar and molar areas are more commonly involved.

A5.15   (a) 5| is a macrodont. A similar effect is sometimes seen when the head moves slightly during the taking of a pantomograph but, in such instances, a similar disturbance occurs in all structures through which the X-ray beam is passing at the time of the head movement. In this instance the upper second premolar would also be distorted and usually there would be a step in the lower border of the right mandible.

(b) This is a particularly obvious but normal anterior nasal spine.

FURTHER READING

Banks, P. (1983). *Killey's Fractures of the Mandible* (3rd edn). Wright PSG, Bristol.

Banks, P. (1987). *Killey's Fractures of the Middle Third of the Facial Skeleton* (5th edn). Wright PSG, Bristol.

Bydder, G. M. (1986). Magnetic resonance imaging of the central nervous system. In *Recent Advances in Radiology and Medical Imaging* (ed R. E. Steines and R. Sherwood) Vol 8, pp. 45–60. Churchill Livingstone, Edinburgh and London.

Cawson, R. A. and Eveson, J. W. (1987). *Oral Pathology and diagnosis: Colour Atlas with Integrated Text.* Heinemann Medical, London.

Donlon, W. C. and Moon, K. L. (1987). Comparison of magnetic resonance imaging, arthrotomography and clinical and surgical findings in temporomandibular joint internal derangements. *Oral Surg., Oral Med., Oral Path.* 64, 2–5.

Foster, T. D. (1982). *A Textbook of Orthodontics.* Blackwell Scientific, Oxford.

Freedman, M. (ed). (1988). *Clinical Imaging,* pp. 2–45. Churchill Livingstone, New York, Edinburgh.

Graft, B. M. and Sickles, E. (1986). A cost analysis comparing xeroradiography to film technics for intraoral radiography. *J Publ. Hlth Dent.* 46, 96–105.

Graft, B. M, White, S. C. and Bauer, J. G. (1988). A clinical comparison between xeroradiography and film radiography for the detection of recurrent caries. *Oral Surg., Oral Med., Oral Path.,* 65, 483–9.

Henderson, D. (1985). *Orthognathic Surgery.* Wolfe Medical, London.

Isherwood, I. and Jenkins, P. R. (1987), MRI—the body. In *A Textbook of Radiology and Imaging* (ed. D. Sutton), pp. 1810–49. Churchill Livingstone, Edinburgh and London.

Jones, J. H. and Mason, D. K. (eds). (1990). *Oral Manifestations of Systemic Disease* (2nd edn). Balliere Tindall, London.

Juniper, R. P. (1987). The pathogenesis and investigation of TMJ dysfunction. *Br. J. Oral Maxillofac. Surg.,* 25, 105–12.

Killey, H. C. and Kay, L. W. (1975). *The Maxillary Sinus and its Dental Implications.* Wright PSG, Bristol.

Laurell, K. A., Tootle, R., Cunningham, R., Beltram, J. and Simon, S. (1987). Magnetic resonance imaging of the temporomandibular joint. Part I: Literature review. *J. Prosth. Dent.* 58, 83–9.

Laurell, K. A., Tootle, R., Cunningham, R., Beltram, J. and Simon, S. (1987). Magnetic resonance imaging of the temporomandibular joint. Part II: Comparison with laminographic, autopsy and histological findings. *J. Prosth. Dent.* 58, 211–18.

Lloyd, G. A. S. (1987). The paranasal sinuses. In *A Textbook of Radiology and Imaging* (ed. D. Sutton), pp. 1285–98. Churchill Livingstone, Edinburgh and London.

Lloyd, G. A. S. and Sutherland, G. R. (1987). The orbit and eye. In *A Textbook of Radiology and Imaging* (ed. D. Sutton), pp. 1315–41. Churchill Livingstone, Edinburgh and London.

Lucas, R. B. (1984). *Pathology of Tumours of the Oral Tissues.* Churchill Livingstone, Edinburgh and London.

Mason, D. K. and Chisholm, D. M. (1975). *Salivary Glands in Health and Disease.* W. B. Saunders, London.

Partridge, M., Langdon, J. D., Borthwick-Clark, A. and Rankin, S. (1986). Diagnostic techniques for parotid disease. *Br. J. Oral Maxillofac. Surg.* 24, 311–22.

Pitts, N. B. (1983). Monitoring of caries progression in permanent and primary posterior approximal enamel by bitewing radiography. *Community Dent. Oral Epidemiol.* 11, 228–35.

Porter, S. R., Porter, K. M. and Scully, C. (1989). Special tests. In *The Dental Patient* (ed. C. Scully), pp. 63–103. Heinemann Medical, Oxford.

Rafto, S. E. and Gefter, W. B. (1988). MRI of the upper aerodigestive tract and neck. *Radiol. Clinics N. Amer.* 26, 547–71.

Renton, P. (1987). Teeth and jaws. In *A Textbook of Radiology and Imaging* (ed. D. Sutton), pp. 1342–72. Churchill Livingstone, Edinburgh and London.

Rhys Davies, E. (1987). Radioisotope imaging. In *A Textbook of Radiology and Imaging* (ed. D. Sutton), pp. 1739–72. Churchill Livingstone, Edinburgh and London.

Scully, C. (1986). Sjögren's syndrome: clinical and laboratory features, immunopathogenesis and management. *Oral Surg., Oral Med., Oral Path.* 62, 510–23.

Scully, C. (1989). *Patent Care: A Dental Surgeon's Guide.* British Dental Journal, London.

Scully, C. and Cawson, R. A. (1987). *Medical Problems in Dentistry* (2nd edn). Wright, Bristol.

Scully, C. and Flint, S. R. (1989). *Atlas of Stomatology.* Dunitz, London.

Shear, M. (1983). *Cysts of the Oral Regions* (2nd edn). Wright PSG, Bristol.

Soames, J. V. and Southam, J. C. (1985). *Oral Pathology.* Oxford University Press, Oxford.

Stephens, C. D. and Isaacson, K. G. (1990). *Exercises in Orthodontic Assessment.* Heinemann Medical, Oxford.

White, S. C., Graft, B. M. and Bauer, J. G. (1988). A clinical comparison of xeroradiography and film radiography for the detection of proximal caries. *Oral Surg., Oral Med., Oral Path.* 65, 2–8.

Wilson, N. H. F. (1987). Dental xeroradiography. In *Dental Annual* (ed. D. Derrick), pp. 261–71. Wright PSG, Bristol.

Wolf, J., Jarvinen, H. J. and Hietanen, J. (1986). Gardner's dento-maxillary stigmas in patients with familial adenomatosis coli. *Br. J. Oral Maxillofac. Surg.* 24, 410–16.

SUBJECT INDEX